59

W9-AYV-477

Basic Shiatsu

By Michio Kushi
and Edward Esko

Foreword by Michael Joutras

615.82
K97

One Peaceful World Press
Becket, Massachusetts

Note to the Reader:

It is advisable for the reader to seek the guidance of a physician and appropriate healthcare professional before implementing the approach to health suggested by this book. It is essential that any reader who has any reason to suspect a serious illness, who is pregnant, or has another condition that requires special care or consideration, contact a physician for guidance and advice about the suitability of the material contained herein. Neither this nor any other book should be used a susbstitute for professional medical care or treatment.

Basic Shiatsu
© 1995 by Michio Kushi and Edward Esko

All rights reserved. Printed in the United States of America. No part of this book may be used or reproduced in any manner whatsoever without written permission except in the case of brief quotations embodied in critical articles or reviews. For information, contact the publisher.

For further information on mail-order sales, wholesale or retail discounts, distribution, translations, and foreign rights, please contact the publisher:

One Peaceful World Press
P.O. Box 10
Leland Road
Becket, MA 01223
U.S.A.

Telephone (413) 623-2322
Fax (413) 623-8827

First Edition: May 1995
10 9 8 7 6 5 4 3 2

ISBN 1–882984–10–2
Printed in U.S.A.

Contents

Foreword

Shiatsu has become one of the most popular forms of natural healthcare in the last few decades. This ancient healing art is being rediscovered at an important time for society—when people's health and well-being are declining rapidly in the modern world.

Many are searching for alternative means of improving and maintaining their health. Shiatsu is both therapeutic and preventive, enhancing the body's self-healing ability for a variety of ailments and also strengthening it to avoid imbalances from arising. I hope that this book will stimulate your interest in studying this fascinating therapy and by attending classes or seminars on Shiatsu.

After many years of being a Shiatsu practitioner, I'm still amazed at its power to help change sickness to health, sadness to joy, stress to relaxation, pain to ease. Shiatsu is as much fun to give as it is to receive, and a valuable learning experience for giver and receiver. Please enjoy this wonderful way of helping others to become healthier and happier.

Michael Anthony Joutras
Becket, Massachusetts
February 10, 1995

Michael Anthony Joutras teaches Shiatsu at the Kushi Institute in Becket, Massachusetts.

Introduction

Massage is one of the most important elements of macrobiotic and holistic healing. Like acupuncture, it involves stimulating and unblocking the invisible pathways which channel energy throughout the body. Energy becomes blocked or stagnated through accumulation of mucus, fats, or toxins in the blood, organs, or joints, which in turn causes stiffness or pain. Blockages and accumulations are caused by dietary imbalances and a lack of proper activity. They interfere with the flow of energy and contribute to illness.

Basic massage uses only the hands and fingertips and can be learned in several hours. With practice, the student can develop his or her ability and make massage into a comprehensive and effective healing art. It can be done almost anytime and anywhere.

The style of massage presented in this book is based on an understanding of the energy constitution of the body, and the interconnectedness of all of its parts and functions. *Shiatsu*, or "finger-pressure," deals with underlying energy imbalances and helps improve overall vitality and conductivity to the forces of heaven and earth. In this way, it helps activate overall vitality and conductivity to environmental energy.

Making your energy harmonious with that of the person you are treating is an intrinsic element of massage. It is therefore important to remember that the physical condition of the practitioner is a key factor in its success. Someone who is healthy, eats a diet of whole grains and vegetables, and who radiates a calm and vibrant energy will transfer this to the person who is receiving the massage.

A Word About Energy

Thousands of years ago, people understood that the human body was made up of something else besides skin, bones, cells, and fluids. They understood that an invisible or undetectable force permeated everything, from stars to atoms, from grains of sand to grains of rice. We can think of this invisible quality as the energy of life itself.

This invisible force was given names such as *Ki* in Japan, *Ch'i* in China, and *prana* in India. These terms are still in use today, as are arts based on the use of this energy. In acupuncture, for example, thin metal needles are used to adjust energy and establish balance or health. The acupuncturist will use his needles to channel energy to places that lack it, or from places that have too much.

The healing traditions of India, China, and Japan are based on the understanding and use of energy. Ayurveda, the traditional medicine of India, which dates back at least 5,000 years, taught that all things are appearances of universal consciousness or energy. According to the centuries-old philosophy of Oriental medicine, first recorded in China in *The Yellow Emperor's Classic of Internal Medicine*, life energy takes countless forms, including mind and body, spirit and matter, heaven and earth. All things are different appearances of universal energy.

The understanding of energy is basic to the Eastern concept of health and healing. In Japan, for example, sickness is described as *Byo-Ki*, or "suffering energy." Kahuna medicine, the native healing tradition of Hawaii, is based on the same understanding. The Kahuna word for good health means "abundance of energy." Poor health is understood to result from either a weakness, or lack of energy, or from blockage or stagnation of energy in the body. The Kahuna word for "healing" means to restore energy and achieve a condition of harmony or fullness.

Energy flows through the body along clearly defined channels. The body as a whole, including all of its cells, organs, and tissues, can be visualized as a complex network of energy. Energy flows through the body in the same way that water flows from a river into many small streams. The primary channel of

8

energy runs from the top of the head to the sexual organs. This central meridian runs deep within the body and is the main source of life energy.

Energy moves along the primary channel in two main directions: downward from heaven to earth (yang energy), and upward from earth to heaven (yin energy). Heaven's yang energy originates in the cosmos, and spirals in toward the center of the earth. Earth's yin force is produced by the rotation of the planet and spirals up from the earth's surface.

There are seven focal points of energy located along the primary channel. In ancient India, these highly charged energy centers were named *chakras*, or spiral "wheels." The chakras are like radiating suns that supply energy to the body, charging and vitalizing all of its functions. The strong charge of energy in the chakras and along the primary channel radiates out toward the periphery of the body, in the same way that energy radiates out from the center of a pumpkin and forms lines or ridges at the surface. These surface lines are known as *meridians*, or energy channels.

The meridians run just below the skin. They send shoots, or branches, up toward the surface of the skin and also branch inside toward the inner regions of the body. The upward shoots end in small holes, or openings, at the surface of the body through which energy from the outside enters and through which energy from inside the body is discharged. These openings are usually referred to as *points*, and there are several hundred major ones along the meridian network. The inner branches continuously divide into smaller and smaller branches, each of which is connected to a cell. Each living cell thus receives energy from the meridians, chakras, and primary channel. Each cell is part of this invisible network. To be alive means to be charged by life energy.

Yin and Yang

The movement of energy in the body is governed by the same rhythm we see in nature. The tides ebb and flow, the moon waxes and wanes, the sun rises and sets. Water flows downhill and condenses into lakes and oceans, then evaporates and rises into the atmosphere. This up and down, expanding and contracting, inward and outward rhythm is found everywhere. The human body is no exception. The structure of the body is based on complementary polarity. Some parts are hard and condensed, while others are soft and expanded. We have a right and a left side, a front and a back, and a condensed central region and an expanded periphery. Certain parts are smaller, others larger.

Energy is continually cycling back and forth between these opposite poles. For example, earth's yin, upward energy is stronger on the right side of the body; while heaven's downward force is stronger on the left. In the morning, earth's energy is predominant, while in the afternoon and evening, heaven's force becomes stronger. Energy is always moving from center to periphery and periphery to center, from front to back and back to front, and from the upper body to the lower body and back again.

Table 1: Yin and Yang in the Body

Yin (expansive energy)	Yang (contractive energy)
Expanded structures	Contracted structures
Peripheral regions	Central regions
Energetic functions	Physical structures
Upper body	Lower body
Loose or soft parts	Tight or hard parts
Moist areas	Dry areas
Smooth surfaces	Rough surfaces
Front	Back
Skin	Muscles, organs, bones
Hollow organs	Solid or compact organs
Colder regions	Warmer regions
Right side	Left side
Flexible parts	Rigid parts

In the Orient, these opposite poles were given the names yin and yang. The term *yin* denotes expanding force or movement, and *yang*, contracting force or movement. In the above table are examples of the way yin and yang appear in the body. The characteristics on the left are examples of yin, expanding energy; those on the right illustrate yang, contracting force.

The goal of Shiatsu is to balance or harmonize the energy of the person we are treating. The principle behind this is quite simple. For example, if a certain part of the body is tense and tight, we can use Shiatsu to soften and relax it. If the energy in a certain part of the body is weak or underactive, Shiatsu can help us activate and energize it.

Health can be defined as a dynamic state of balance in which our energy is neither overactive nor underactive, excessive nor deficient. It is also the state in which our physical condition is not too tight or rigid, nor too loose or expanded. Shiatsu is a direct and powerful tool for adjusting energy and moderating extremes. When someone receives a good massage, he or she will feel refreshed, relaxed, and energized. Excess will have been discharged, weakness will have been strengthened, and tension will have been released. In this fast-paced and stressful world, basic Shiatsu can help everyone achieve greater health and well-being.

Organ-Pairs and Meridian Flow

The organs of the body develop in pairs. Yin organs have a hollow structure and an active or yang flow of energy along their corresponding meridian. Examples include the large intestine, small intestine, gallbladder, and stomach. Yang organs have a dense, compact structure and a more yin, subtle meridian flow. Examples include the lungs, heart, liver, and spleen. Yin organs are paired with yang organs. The organ-pairs complement and make balance with each other. Their functions are intimately related. Imbalance in one is a sign of imbalance in the other. Treating an organ with Shiatsu produces an immediate effect in its complementary partner. The organ-pairs were first recorded thousands of years ago in *The Yellow Emperor's Classic*, and are shown in the following table.

11

Table 2: Classification of Organs According to Structure

Yang (solid and compact) Organs	Yin (hollow and expanded) Organs
Lungs	Large intestine
Heart	Small intestine
Liver	Gallbladder
Spleen (pancreas)	Stomach
Kidney	Bladder
Heart governor function	Triple heater function

In addition to five pairs of organs, Oriental philosopher-healers identified two comprehensive body functions that are produced by energetic activity in the chakras, especially the heart, stomach, and small intestine chakras. The chakras generate and supply life energy to the body as a whole. Their functions affect, but are not limited to, the activity of individual organs. Energy converging toward the chakras drives the rhythm of the heart and the movements of digestion and absorption, including the absorption of nutrients by the small intestine and water by the large intestine. The convergence of energy in these chakras therefore influences the circulation of blood, lymph, and other bodily fluids. This comprehensive function is referred to in Oriental medicine as the *heart governor*.

The chakras also convert energy from the environment into the internal heat and energy required for life. This energy is supplied to all of the body's cells. The chakras are the source of the power that drives the metabolic functions of every cell, including cell growth and the conversion of nutrients to energy. This body-wide function is referred to in Oriental medicine as the *triple heater*.

Like opposite electric charges, yin and yang provide the impetus for the movement of energy throughout the body. Each organ is part of a meridian, and the meridians are all connected in a continuous cycle of energy. The meridians themselves can be thought of as the .yin, peripheral energetic component of the body's energy system, and the organs, as the yang, central physical part of this system. Energy flows from the center of the body to the periphery, and from the periphery back to the center. The fingers and toes are the most peripheral parts of the meridians, and correspond to the organs deep inside. The flow through these channels is continuous and unbroken.

In Shiatsu, we make use of all twelve meridians, in addition to two others that correspond directly to the primary channel and chakras. One, known as the *conception vessel*, runs up the front of the body in the center. The other, known as the *governing vessel*, runs up the center of the spine.

The meridians are an integral part of the overall functioning of each organ. Changes in the organs produce corresponding changes in the meridians. Stimulating the points and meridians influences the condition of the organs. This relationship makes it possible to diagnose or evaluate the organs by means of the points and meridians. It also makes it possible to use the points and meridians to treat the organs. The complementary-antagonistic relationship existing between the center and periphery, and between the body's physical structures and invisible energy pathways, provides the basis for the effectiveness of Shiatsu and other Oriental therapies.

Giving a Balanced Massage

The basic full-body massage can be simplified in five steps: (1) the shoulders, neck, and head; (2) the back; (3) the arms and hands; (4) the legs and feet; and (5) the face and front of the body. To these we have added: (6) techniques for concluding the massage; (7) guidelines for evaluating the receiver's condition and offering dietary and lifestyle advice; and (8) suggestions for developing your own natural healing ability.

The basic massage routine presented in this book needs to be adapted to each person's unique condition. If, for example, a person is experiencing pain or severe rigidity in the joints or in any other part of the body, it is advisable to omit

13

the procedures that call for massaging these areas. You can try the full body massage presented below, one step at a time, or can try only parts of it.

Table 3 : Yin and Yang in Shiatsu

Yin Techniques	Yang Techniques
Using light or superficial pressure	Using firm or deep pressure
Stroking or brushing	Pounding or tapping
Rubbing or kneading	Pressing
Massaging from center to periphery	Massaging from periphery to center
Focusing on your inhalation	Focusing on your exhalation
Rotation in a clockwise direction	Rotation in a counterclockwise direction
Breaking contact with receiver	Making contact with receiver
Pausing	Acting
Releasing tension	Generating tension
Dispersing energy	Focusing energy
Pulling	Pushing
Adopting a slower pace	Adopting a rapid pace
Using your palms	Using your thumbs or fingertips
Massaging a wide area	Pressing specific points
Massaging the periphery or front of the body	Massaging the center or back of the body

Also, unlike other forms of massage, Shiatsu does not require the removal of clothing or the use of oils. Loose-fitting cotton clothing is best for giving and receiving massage. The massage can also be performed simply on blankets or cushions placed on the floor. All you need is a quiet and undisturbed space. Each time you give Shiatsu, there are a variety of yin and yang techniques you can use to adjust the balance of the massage, and these are shown in the above table.

A balanced massage incorporates the energies of yang

and yin in the form of fast and slow movements, firm and gentle pressure, breathing out and breathing in, activating and calming effects. The more you practice, the easier it will be for you to apply yin and yang in a spontaneous and intuitive manner, so that your technique is at all times appropriate to each person's unique condition and needs. As your skill increases, you begin to serve as a clear channel for the energies of heaven and earth, which are the ultimate sources of health and healing.

Step 1
Massaging the Head and Shoulders

If the shoulders are tight, swollen, and painful when pressed, energy is not flowing smoothly through the body. A person in this condition has difficulty relaxing and is frequently tired. Tight shoulders are also a sign of stagnation in the intestines that blocks the active flow of energy in the lower body.

To help relieve shoulder tension, release intestinal stagnation, and vitalize the body as a whole:

1. Ask the receiver to sit comfortably on a blanket or cushions with his or her spine straight and shoulders and arms relaxed. Keeping your spine straight, kneel behind the receiver. Extend your arms forward and grasp both shoulders with a firm but gentle pressure. Keep your hands in this position and begin to harmonize your energies by breathing together.

Heaven's force charges your left hand and the receiver's left shoulder; earth's force, your right hand and the receiver's right shoulder. Placing your hands on the shoulders harmonizes these energies and helps the receiver to relax. With your hands in this position, breathe together for about a minute. Breathing in a calm and relaxed manner also centers your energy, making you better able to give massage.

Throughout the massage, keep your breathing steady and even. Center your breathing in the lower abdomen, or hara. This stabilizes your energy and enables you to move more freely.

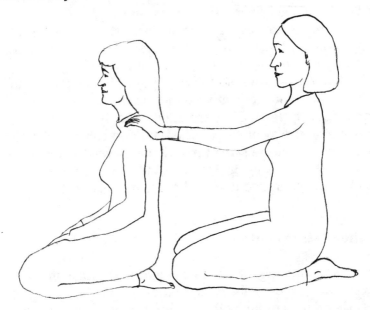

2. Begin to massage the shoulders with a kneading motion. Start with the area closest to the neck and gradually work outward toward the tips of the shoulders. Repeat several times.

3. Stand up behind the receiver. Keeping your thumbs straight, press with the tips of both thumbs along the top of the shoulder muscles on both sides of the neck. Gently push in, and then quickly release the pressure. Begin from the innermost region on both sides of the neck, and work outward toward the tips of the shoulders. This procedure activates the intestines and helps release stagnated energy.

When performing this part of the massage, coordinate your breathing with that of the receiver. To do this properly, inhale together, and as you breathe out, press downward. Press along the shoulder muscle several times before proceeding to the next step of the massage.

4. With your hands in the position indicated in step one, extend your middle fingers down the front of the body to massage the area under the collarbone on both sides. Using

the tips of the fingers, massage for about one minute. If this area is painful or overly sensitive, the lungs are overly expanded from mucus deposits, liquids, and sugar.

This region corresponds to an important point on the lung meridian, Lung 1, or *Chu-Fu*. Refer to the chart of the lung meridian for the precise location of this point.

5. Keeping your wrists loose and flexible, use the outside edge of your hands to gently pound the shoulders by rapidly alternating between the left and right hand. Begin at the neck and work your way outward. The shoulders can be done separately or both at the same time. Repeat several times. After finishing step five, again massage the shoulders as in step two. The shoulders should now be soft and relaxed.

Further Refinements

Trace the pathways of the large intestine, small intestine, triple heater, and gallbladder meridians on the shoulders. Massage each meridian with your thumbs and fingertips during step two. Use your thumbs to press and massage meridian points on the shoulders.

Neck

Tension or stiffness in the neck is a common problem today, aggravated by the excessive intake of protein, saturated fat, sugar, refined foods, and by overeating and over-drinking in general.

When the neck becomes stiff, energy does not flow smoothly through the small intestine, large intestine, stomach, bladder, and gallbladder meridians, all of which run along the neck. Stiffness in the neck also indicates diminished physical and mental flexibility, including a reduced capacity for natural, spontaneous expression and enjoyment.

To help relieve tension in the neck and stimulate the organs and meridians:

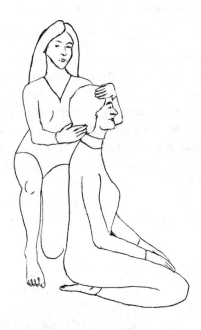

1. Shift your position so that you are sitting behind the receiver at a 45-degree angle. Place the bulk of your weight on one knee and raise your other leg so that your foot is on the floor. If you are right-handed, shift to the left, so that you can use your left hand to support the receiver's forehead, while leaving your right hand free to massage the back of the neck. Persons who are left-handed should shift in the opposite direction, leaving the left hand free for the neck massage.

2. Tilt the receiver's head slightly backward, and place the tips of your thumb and middle finger in the indented places at the base of the skull on both sides of the back of the neck. Massage this region for about a minute or until hardness or tension is relieved. Pain in this area frequently indicates that the receiver is eating too many fatty foods, which interfere with the smooth functioning of the liver and gallbladder.

Massaging these points (Gallbladder 20, or *Fu-Chi*) on either side of the neck releases tension in the head, neck, and shoulders. These points were traditionally used to relieve such conditions as headache, including migraine, influenza, hypertension, ringing in the ears, eye strain, and dizziness. Refer to the chart of the gallbladder meridian for the location of these points.

3. Return the receiver's head to the normal angle, and beginning from the above points, use the tip of your thumb and middle finger to massage in a straight line down the back of the neck to the base, generally along the path of the gallbladder meridian. Use a deep but gentle pinching motion in which you knead and stimulate the neck muscle with your fingertips. Repeat several times, making sure to loosen any hardness or tension.

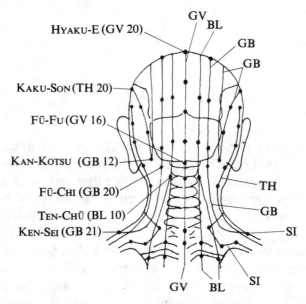

4. Place the tip of your thumb in the center of the neck at the base of the skull. This region corresponds to a point known as *Fu-Fu* (Governing Vessel 16). Begin breathing together, and after several breaths, tilt the head back, as in step two, and on the final inhalation, push your thumb inward and upward into the point, lifting the head slightly upward. Use your supporting hand to help lift the head. At the peak of the inhalation, vibrate your thumb for several seconds, and as you breathe out, release the pressure and allow the head to return to its normal position. Repeat several times.

This procedure releases stagnation in the liver and relaxes the neck and shoulders. This point was traditionally used to treat conditions such as headache, nervousness, hypertension, dizziness, and mucus in the sinuses or nasal cavities.

5. Return to your original position behind the receiver. Place your right hand firmly on the shoulder, resting the inside of the hand against the neck for support. With your left hand on the left side of the head, begin to rotate the head slowly toward the right in a clockwise direction. (This helps relax tension in the neck and shoulders.)

As much as possible, allow the head to rotate itself; it is better to use your hands only to support and guide the rotation. After a minute, reverse your hands and begin to rotate in the opposite, counterclockwise direction. (This helps to stabilize energy in the person's body.) Continue for about one minute.

Further Refinements

Use your supporting hand to tilt the head to one side, and with the thumb of your free hand, press down the gallbladder and bladder meridians on the opposite side from the base of the skull to shoulder. Reverse your hands and do the same on the other side of the neck. Then use your thumb to press down the governing vessel meridian from the base of the skull to the top of the spine.

Locate and massage important points on the neck, including *Ten-Chu*, or Bladder 10. This point was traditionally used to relieve a variety of disorders, including headaches, insomnia, nervousness, tightness in the neck or shoulder muscles, hysteria, eye diseases, sore throats, and stuffy nose.

Head

In the human body and throughout nature, the part reflects the whole. This is especially true in the relationship between the head and the rest of the body, since there are areas on the head that relate to all of the major organs and body functions, including the chakras.

To stimulate these areas and their corresponding organs and functions, and energize the body as a whole:

1. Stand up behind the receiver. Place your fingers on either side of his or her head and extend your thumbs so that they are free to massage the central part of the top of the head. Place your thumbs behind each other, and press down in a straight line extending from the hairline back across the top of the head and down the back of the head to the base of the skull. Repeat several times. Massaging this line, which corresponds to the governing vessel meridian, energizes and vitalizes the entire body.

2. Directly on top of the head in the center is a point on the governing vessel meridian known as the "hundred meeting point" (Governing Vessel 20, or *Hyaku-E.*) Energy from the entire body gathers there.

Place your fingers on either side of the receiver's head and position your thumbs just above the point. Breathe together several times, and at the peak of the final exhalation, press the hundred meeting point. While applying pressure, vibrate your thumbs for several seconds and then release. This helps to release energy that has become stagnant anywhere in the body. Repeat several times. This point was traditionally used to ease the symptoms of headache, nervousness, hypertension, stuffy nose, insomnia, and constipation.

3. Locate the receiver's hair spiral. Position your hands as in step two, breathe together, and press your thumbs into the center of the spiral, using the same methods as above. Release and repeat several times. The hair spiral is the place where heaven's force enters the body, and from here, flows down along the primary channel. Massaging the hair spiral helps to energize and vitalize energy in the chakras and body as a whole.

4. Visualize parallel lines running on either side of the governing vessel meridian, each about two finger-widths from this central line, from the hairline to the base of the skull. These correspond to the bladder meridian. Using your thumbs, press down both lines simultaneously. Extend your

fingertips down the sides of the head for support.

5. Visualize another set of parallel lines running about two finger-widths out from the bladder lines explained above. Using the same technique presented in step four, massage these lines from the hairline to the base of the skull.

6. Use your thumbs to massage the sides of the head, beginning at the hairline and working your way around to the back of the head. Place your free hand on the opposite side of the head for support. Do one side and then the other.

7. Extend your fingers down the sides of the head, and with your middle fingers, massage both temples simultaneously, using a slow, upward circular motion. Continue for about a minute or until all tension in this area is released.

8. Use your thumbs to massage in a semi-circle on the sides of the head around the ears, beginning at the region of the temple and working around to the base of the skull. Do one side and then the other.

9. Grasp both ears with thumbs and middle fingers. Begin to massage the ears by pulling them gently upward from the top, outward from the side, and then downward from the lobe. Repeat several times, allowing your fingers to slide across the inner portion of the ear to the edge. The ears correlate with the kidneys, and this part of the massage is good for loosening stagnation in these organs and improving circulation and vitality.

10. Using your fingertips, gently pound the top of the head, making sure to keep your wrists loose and flexible. You can also tighten your hands into a fist and gently pound the head with your knuckles. Be sure to stimulate the entire head, including the top, sides, and back. Do each region for about thirty seconds.

After finishing this part of the massage, sit down behind the receiver and again knead the shoulders as explained previously. If the massage has been done properly, the shoulders should be soft and relaxed, meaning that energy in the primary channel, chakras, and meridians is now smooth and active.

Further Refinements

Trace the pathways of the gallbladder and triple heater meridians on the side of the head. Use your thumbs to press along these meridians, beginning from the front of the ear and working your way up and around toward the back of the head. Study, confirm, and use important points on the sides of the head and around the ear.

Step 2
Massaging the Back

Massaging the back stimulates all of the major organs. This is accomplished by massaging the bladder meridian (running along either side of the spine), the chakras, and the roots of the autonomic nerve branches (radiating outward from the spinal cord to the internal organs). The bladder meridian includes points, known in Japanese as *Yu* points, where energy enters the body and charges each of the major organs. The Yu points are found in pairs on either side of the spine. When massaging the meridians, you can either massage in their general vicinity, or consult the diagrams at the back of the book for their locations.

To massage the back:

1. Have the receiver lie on his or her stomach, the head turned sideways and arms extended comfortably to the side. Place a pillow or cushion under the receiver's head so that he or she is comfortable.

2. Kneel alongside the receiver so that one hand is free to massage the entire back. If you are right-handed, sit on their left; vice versa if you are left- handed. Place your hand so that the center of the palm rests lightly on the spine. Slowly brush down the spine to the buttocks, as if you were smoothing energy downward.

3. Place one palm on the spine, and place your other hand on top of it. Starting at the upper spine, breathe together, and as you exhale, gently press downward. Add your body weight by leaning forward as you press. Release pres-

ᵤ the next inhalation, and repeat down the length
ᵧine to the tail bone.

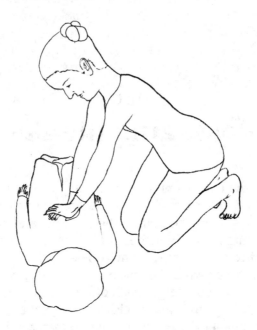

4. To massage the governing vessel meridian running
along the center of the spine (which energizes the chakras),
insert your thumbs one below the other in the indented spaces between the vertebrae. Extend your fingers outward and
place them on the rib cage for support. Begin at the top of the
spine. Breathe together and on the exhalation gently push
your thumbs downward, releasing pressure on the following
inhalation. Insert your thumbs in the next set of spaces and
repeat down the entire length of the spine.

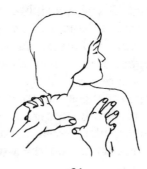

5. Hold your fingers firmly together and extend them outward. Insert your fingertips in the indented area on either side of the spine. Beginning at the upper spine, move your hand rapidly in a cutting or sawing motion. Work your way down the entire length of the spine, using this indented area as a pathway. Do the same thing on the opposite side of the spine. This releases muscle tension in the back as a whole.

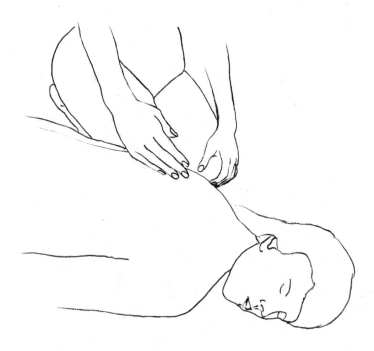

6. Find the inner set of bladder meridians which run along two parallel lines located about two finger-widths out from the center of the spine. Using the technique described above, press your thumbs along the length of the meridian, beginning at the shoulders and proceeding down the back and across the buttocks in one-inch steps.

When massaging the rib cage, insert your thumbs in the spaces between the ribs. This procedure is particularly effective when you coordinate your breathing with that of the receiver, by deeply breathing in and deeply exhaling in the same rhythm. In this part of the massage, you are using the Yu points to stimulate the internal organs.

7. Find the outer set of bladder meridians which run along two parallel lines about two finger-widths out from the inner set of meridians. Use the above technique to massage both sides simultaneously, from the shoulders to the buttocks.

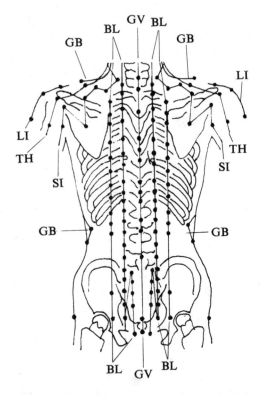

8. Use the fingertips, thumb, and base of the palm to massage the receiver's shoulder blade. Continue with active massage for about one minute, loosening any tension in the surrounding muscles and tendons. Repeat with the other shoulder blade. This procedure activates the lungs.

9. Place your thumb in the center of the shoulder blade. Breathe together with the receiver, and press as you exhale, massaging this area with a quick circular motion. Repeat three times and proceed to the other shoulder blade. Rotate

your thumb counterclockwise to send energy; clockwise to release energy from the receiver's body.

This point, known as *Ten-So*, or Small Intestine 11, activates and releases tension in the small intestine. It was used by Oriental doctors to relieve chest pain, neck and shoulder stiffness, pleurisy, and breast pain. It was also used to treat the inability to produce breast milk, disorders of the liver and gallbladder, and lack of strength in the arms.

10. Place both hands together across the spine in the region of the waist. Place your thumbs on one side, and your fingers on the other side of the spine. Use a deep kneading motion to massage this area. Pain here is a sign of expansion or tightness in the kidneys, and indicates potential weakening of overall vitality. This procedure loosens stagnation in the kidneys and adrenal glands.

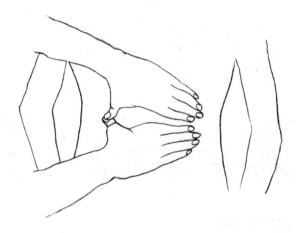

11. Use your palm, fingers, and thumb to knead and rub the entire back, relieving any tension or stagnation in the muscles and along the meridians. Start at the upper region and massage down the periphery of the back, one side at a time. Use your left hand to send energy to the receiver; your right hand to draw energy from the receiver's body. After you finish, use both hands to smooth energy down the spine and both sides of the back.

12. To massage the buttocks, move slightly downward so

that you can reach the indented area in the center of both sides of the buttock. Push the base of your palms firmly in this area and then massage with an upward and outward circular motion. Repeat for about one minute. This is especially good for activating the organs in the lower body and strengthening overall vitality.

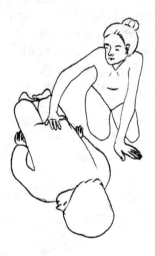

Then, place your hand on the tail bone. Use the base of your palm to gently pound the tail bone. Continue for about thirty seconds, in order to send stimulation along the entire length of the spine. This procedure also helps strengthen sexual vitality.

Further Refinements

Study and confirm the location of the Yu points along the bladder meridian. Use these points to stimulate the organs when you massage down the bladder meridian.

Step 3
Massaging the Arms and Hands

Six meridians run along the arm. Three—the lung, heart governor (the comprehensive function responsible for the circulation of blood and body fluids), and heart—run down the inside of the arm from the armpit to the hand, and out to the fingers. The other three—the large intestine, triple heater (the body-wide function responsible for the generation of heat and caloric energy), and small intestine—run from the fingers up the outside of the arm to the shoulder.

During this part of the massage, the receiver can continue lying comfortably on his front. If he is uncomfortable in this position, he can turn over and lie on his back. This part of the massage can be performed with the receiver in either position. It can also be done with the receiver sitting up. To massage the arms and hands:

1. Place your hand on the root of the arm with your thumb inserted in the person's armpit and your fingers placed across the top of the shoulder joint. Grasp the wrist with your other hand and stretch the arm by pushing your hand down and gently pulling the arm outward with your other hand. Repeat several times. (*See illustration next page.*)

2. Grasp the arm by placing both hands in the area between the wrist and the elbow. Using the shoulder as the axis of rotation, gently twist the entire arm first in one direction and then in the other. Repeat several times

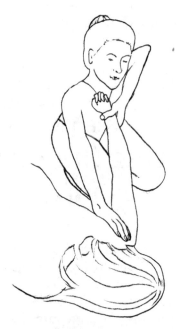

3. Place one hand above and the other below the elbow. Gently twist the upper and lower sections of the arm in opposite directions, as if you were wringing out a wet towel. Repeat by twisting each section in the reverse direction.

4. Use the palm and fingers of your active hand to press down both sides of the arm, making sure to loosen any tension in the muscles and tendons. Work your way down to the hands and fingertips. These four procedures release tension in the muscles and along the meridians. They help prepare the arm for the next part of the massage.

5. Visualize three parallel lines running about two finger-widths apart along the inside of the arm from the armpit to the wrist. These correspond to the heart, heart governor, and lung meridians.

Place one hand under the arm for support, and with the thumb of your other hand, press along each line, starting at the armpit and working your way down to the wrist. Massage the heart meridian (connecting to the little finger), the heart governor (connecting to the middle finger), and then the lung meridian (connecting to the thumb).

As you work your way along each line, spend extra time massaging the elbow and wrist portion with a gentle circular thumb motion. Important points are located in these areas.

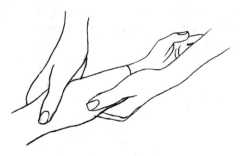

6. As with the above step, visualize three parallel lines running along the outside of the arm, this time in the opposite direction from the wrist to the shoulder. These correspond to the large intestine, triple heater, and small intestine meridians. Using the same technique, massage these outer lines from the wrist to the shoulder.

Start with the large intestine meridian (connecting to the index finger) and proceed to the triple heater (connecting to the ring finger) and small intestine (connecting to the little finger). Pay special attention to the part of each meridian that crosses the elbow and wrist.

7. Support the person's wrist with one hand, and with the other, gently rotate the hand several times. Repeat in the opposite direction. This helps dissolve tension in the wrist, hand, and fingers, and releases stagnation in the meridians.

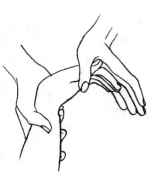

8. Place the hand on one knee for support. Position the little finger of one of your hands between the thumb and index finger of the receiver's hand, and position your other little finger between the ring and little fingers. Using your little fingers for support, massage the palms by rapidly pressing your thumbs one after the other into the palm, working your way around the entire hand.

Place special emphasis on the area adjacent to the thumb which corresponds to the digestive and respiratory organs. Pain or a reddish or bluish color in this area indicate possible swelling or fatty deposits in the lungs and large intestine.

9. Massage the center of both palms. This area, which includes an important point on the heart governor meridian, energizes the heart, stomach, and hara chakras, together with sexual vitality. This point is known as Heart Governor 8, or *Ro-Kyu*. Pain in this point frequently indicates that the circulatory system is overworking, and that the receiver may be experiencing fatigue.

Place one hand under the person's hand for support, and with the thumb of your active hand, press the center of the palm, and then release. To send energy, rotate your thumb in a counterclockwise direction. To release energy, rotate your thumb clockwise. Repeat several times.

This point is used by Oriental doctors to diagnose and treat general fatigue, heart pain, arthritis of the wrists and fingers, jaundice, and nose bleeding.

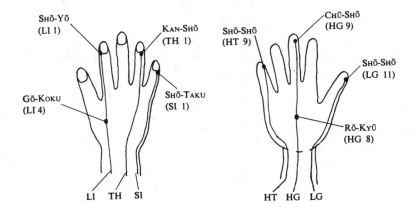

10. Turn the hand so that the outside is exposed. Find the indented area between the thumb and index finger. Massage this area for about one minute, using a deep, circular motion of your thumb to release tension and stagnation. This area is along the large intestine meridian, and corresponds to an important point known as *Go-Koku*, or Large Intestine 4.

Pain or tightness indicate stagnation or overexpansion in the large intestine. This point can be used to diagnose or treat the large intestine. It can also be used to treat headaches, facial disorders, nosebleeds, and epilepsy.

11. Each of the fingers corresponds to one of the meridians that run along the arm, in the following order: thumb — lung; index finger—large intestine; middle finger—heart governor; ring finger—triple heater; little finger (inside)—heart; and little finger (outside)—small intestine.

When massaging the fingers, imagine a series of five points, three located in the center of the three sections of each finger and two located immediately below the finger on the palm. Use four points when massaging the thumb—two in the center of each section and two immediately below in the root of the thumb.

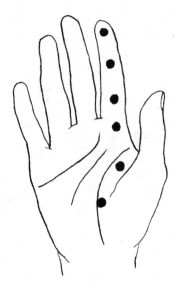

Grasp the wrist with one hand and turn the palm upward. Massage each finger separately by pressing each point with the tip of your thumb, rotating your thumb in a circular motion, releasing, and then proceeding to the next point. Start with the points located at the root of the fingers.

To send energy to the meridians, rotate your thumb counterclockwise; to release energy, rotate your thumb clockwise. Place your fingers on the opposite side of each finger for support. When you reach the last point on the tip of each finger, pull and rotate the finger several times.

12. Use your palm and fingers to brush down both sides of the arm and out through the fingertips. Repeat several times.

Shift to the other side of the receiver and repeat the above steps with the other arm.

Further Refinements

Find the *Go*, *Gen*, and *Sei* points on each meridian. (Refer to diagram at the back of the book.) These points play an important role in regulating the flow of energy. The Go points are located around the elbow and help concentrate and activate energy. Massaging them stimulates the outer regions of the organs.

The Gen, or "source" points are located on or near the wrist and help balance energy. (Go-Koku, or Large Intestine 4, is the Gen point of the large intestine meridian.) The Sei, or "well" points, located on the tips of the fingers, are where Ki pours up and out from the meridians. Massaging the Sei points influences the inner regions of the organs.

You can massage the Go points while you are pressing along the arm meridians. The Gen points can also be massaged at that time or during the hand massage. Massage the Sei points while doing the fingers.

Step 4
Massaging the Legs and Feet

The bladder, gallbladder, and stomach meridians run down along the back, sides, and front of the leg. The kidney, spleen, and liver meridians run up along the inside. Of primary importance when massaging the legs is to activate these meridian pathways, while releasing tension in the legs, feet, and lower body. To massage the legs:

1. Have the receiver lie on his stomach. Shift your position so that you are below his feet. In most cases, you will notice that the legs are not perfectly even. If one leg is longer than the other, this indicates a degree of imbalance between the right and left sides of the body. It may also indicate that the pelvis is slanted in the direction of the longer leg; the result of overexpansion in the organs located on that side, especially the kidneys, intestines, and sexual organs.

To help correct this imbalance, grasp the shorter leg below the ankle. Gently pull the leg slightly upward and outward, lower it to the ground, and then release.

2. Grasp both feet by holding the toes between your palms and fingers. Bend the legs at the knee, cross the feet at the ankles, and press them backward into the buttocks. If the legs and feet are painful or not flexible enough to do this, do not force them.

With the legs in this position, reverse the feet and again

press down into the buttocks. After you finish, return the feet to their normal position on the floor. This stretches and releases stagnation in the meridians.

3. The bladder meridian, which runs down the back, continues down the back of both legs and out to the fifth toe. Using the thumb, press down the meridian from the buttock to the ankle. Each leg may be massaged separately or both at the same time. Use a gentle, penetrating pressure when massaging this meridian; however, ease up when you reach the sensitive area behind the knee, as pressure here can be painful.

If the receiver feels pain when you press the part of the meridian on the center of the calf (corresponding to the large intestine), his or her intestines are overly expanded, and energy in the hara, or small intestine chakra has become weak.

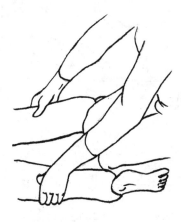

4. When you reach the ankle, locate the point known as *Kon-Ron*, or Bladder 60, on the outside of the ankle near the bone. Massage this point with your middle finger, while placing your thumb on the opposite side of the ankle for support. This point can be used to treat headaches, stiff neck, or disorders in the urinary system.

5. Raise one leg by bending it at the knee. Place one hand below the ankle and grasp the toes with the other. Begin to rotate the foot in a circular motion for about one minute in one direction and then in the other. Do not force the foot to rotate beyond the point at which discomfort is experienced. Pain or

lack of flexibility in the ankles is a sign of hardening of the arteries and joints, and of a general decline in creativity and mental flexibility. This procedure relaxes and energizes the feet and toes.

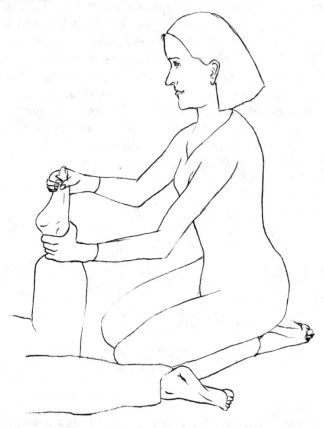

6. With the leg in the above position, use one hand to press the foot downward so that it is parallel to the floor. With the thumb and index finger of your other hand, massage the Achilles tendon by rubbing it vigorously up and down. This tendon correlates to the sexual organs. It should be tight and somewhat firm. If it is loose, the sexual organs may have become weak as a result of dietary excess. Fat around the Achilles tendon suggests fat and mucus deposits in the sexual organs. Massage the Achilles tendon for about thirty seconds. This helps energize sexual vitality.

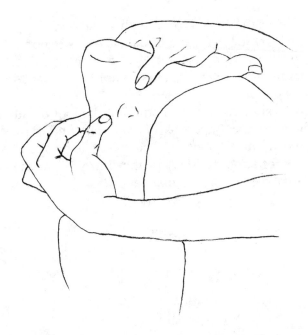

7. Find the point located behind the ankle bone on the inside of the leg. This point, known as *Tai-Kei*, or Kidney 3, can be used to energize the kidneys and bladder. Use the thumb of your free hand to press and massage this point for about thirty seconds.

8. Keeping the foot in the above position, locate the point on the inside of the leg about four finger-widths up from the ankle. Known as *San-In-Ko*, or the "juncture of three yin meridians," this point (Spleen 6) is where the spleen, liver, and kidney meridians intersect.

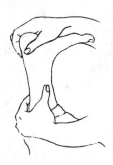

Spleen 6 can be used to strengthen the sexual organs. Use the thumb of your free hand to massage this region for about thirty seconds with a deep but gentle circular motion. **However, please note: this point should not be massaged when a woman is pregnant.**

9. Actively massage the bottom of the foot by alternately pressing with the fingertips of your left and right hands. Place your thumbs opposite to your fingers on the underside of the foot for support. Massage the entire sole of the foot for about thirty seconds in this manner.

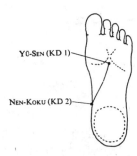

YŪ-SEN (KD 1)

NEN-KOKU (KD 2)

10. On the bottom of the foot, in the indented area about three fingers below the junction of the second and third toes, is an important point on the kidney meridian. Known in Japanese as *Yu-Sen*, or "bubbling spring," this point (Kidney 1) is where the kidney meridian begins its course up the inside of the leg. Place your free hand on the opposite side of the foot for support and press the point with your thumb. You may also vibrate your thumb as you are applying pressure. Release pressure and repeat several times.

If this point is overly sensitive or painful, the kidneys are not functioning at their optimum. To send energy to the kidneys, massage this point in a counterclockwise direction. To release energy from the kidneys, rotate your thumbs in a clockwise direction. Thickening of the skin on the kidney point is caused by the intake of too much animal protein and fat and indicates that energy is not flowing smoothly and the person's vitality is below par.

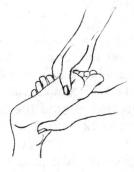

11. Massage the toes by using the pinching technique described for the fingers. As with the fingers, work your way outward to the tip, and then pull and rotate each toe. When you finish each toe, pull excess energy out by gently pulling and snapping the tip.

Each toe corresponds to a particular organ and meridian in the following order: large toe (outside)—spleen; large toe (inside)—liver; second and third toes—stomach; fourth toe—gallbladder; fifth toe—bladder. Each of these organs and their corresponding meridians are stimulated and activated when we massage the toes.

12. Supporting the foot from the underside, use your free hand to rapidly pound the entire bottom of the foot. Tighten your fingers into a fist and pound with the side of your hand. Like the head, palms, ears, and back, the bottoms of the feet have correspondences with the entire body, and the entire body becomes relaxed and energized when we stimulate them.

After you finish the above steps, lower the foot to the floor and repeat steps four through ten with the other foot. After massaging both feet, brush your partner's energy down the back and sides of both legs from the buttocks to the toes.

Further Refinements

Learn the correspondences between certain regions on the bottoms of the feet and the different parts of the body. Use these correspondences when massaging the feet.

The leg meridians also contain Go, Gen, and Sei points. The Go points are located around the knee, the Gen points, around the ankle, and the Sei points, on the toes or bottoms of the feet. Yu-Sen, or Kidney 1, introduced in step nine, is the Sei point of the kidney meridian. Study and use these points during the leg and foot massage.

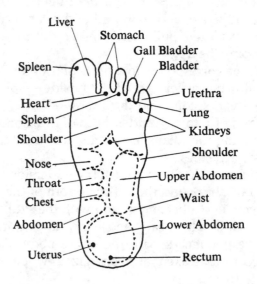

Step 5
Massaging the Front of the Body

Of primary importance when massaging the front of the body is to gently stimulate the organs along with the remaining meridians on the leg. These include the kidney, spleen, and liver meridians which run up the inside of the leg, and the stomach and gallbladder meridians which run down the front side. A simple facial massage can be performed at this time to conclude the basic Shiatsu routine.

To massage the front of the body:

1. Ask the receiver to turn over so that he or she is lying comfortably on the back. Grasp both legs by the ankles and use both hands to generally massage the front and sides of the legs. Begin at the ankles and work up to the pelvis. Try to loosen any tension in the muscles. Repeat several times.

2. Massage the top of the foot by alternately pressing with your thumbs. Place your fingers opposite to your thumbs on the underside of the foot for support. Massage the foot for about thirty seconds in this manner.

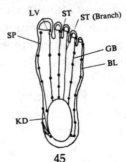

3. Find the liver Gen point located in the indented area between the bones of the first and second toes on the top of the foot. This point is known as *Tai-Sho*, or Liver 3. Massage the point with a deep but gentle circular motion. Massage in a counterclockwise direction to send energy, or in a clockwise direction to release energy.

Massaging this point helps release stagnation in the liver and gallbladder and can be used to treat dizziness and insomnia. After massaging this point on one foot, repeat steps two and three on the other foot.

4. Visualize three parallel lines running up the inside of the leg from the ankle to the pelvis. These correspond to the kidney, spleen, and liver meridians. Place your fingers on the outside of the leg for support, and press upward along each line with your thumbs. Each leg can be massaged separately or both at the same time.

5. As you are massaging the liver meridian, find the point known as *Kyoku-Sen*, or Liver 8, located on the part of the meridian that runs along the knee. Massage this point with a deep but gentle circular motion. This point can be used to activate the liver and gallbladder and to relieve arthritis in the knee, frequent urination, and bladder infection.

6. As you are massaging the spleen meridian, find the point on the inner part of the thigh, about three finger-widths up from the knee, known as *Kek-Kai*, or Spleen 10. Massage this point as above to stimulate the spleen and pancreas.

7. Imagine a line running down the top of the leg on the outside of the knee from the pelvis to the foot. This corresponds to the stomach meridian. Keep your hands in the position described above, only this time, use your fingers to massage down the line and your thumb for support. The legs can be massaged one at a time or simultaneously.

8. The Go point of the stomach meridian is located about three finger-widths below the knee bone. Known as *San-Ri*, or Stomach 36, this point can be used to diagnose or treat stomach disorders and strengthen digestive ability. Locate this point and massage it with your thumb or fingertips for about ten seconds. Often this point will be sensitive to touch.

9. Visualize a line running down the outside of the leg

from the hip socket to the foot. This corresponds to the gall-bladder meridian. Using the above technique, massage down this line also.

As you reach the knee, locate the point known as *Yo-Ryo-Sen*, or Gallbladder 34, located in the indentation on the outside of the leg immediately below the knee. Use your thumbs or fingertips to massage the point. This point was traditionally used to relieve liver, gallbladder, and digestive troubles.

10. Have the receiver raise his or her knees and place the feet flat on the floor. Place your hands on the knees and press the knees upward and then downward toward the abdomen. This helps release tension deep within the intestines. Return the legs to their resting position on the floor.

11. Place the fingers of your active hand together and extend them firmly outward. Place the tips of your extended fingers on the lower right side of the abdomen in the region of the ascending colon. Breathe together and on the exhalation, press gently into the abdomen. Release pressure with the following exhalation, and reposition your hand further up along the ascending colon. Repeat this procedure along the entire length of the colon, moving across the transverse colon and then down the descending colon on the left side.

Pain or hardness in the large intestine is a sign of mucus and fat accumulations, or swelling due to the intake of saturated fats, flour products, sugar, liquid, and overeating in general. This practice can be repeated several times as it is good for promoting regularity in the bowels and releasing stagnation in the lower body.

12. Place your hands across the abdomen. Begin to gently knead and massage the small intestine. Continue for about a minute.

13. Place your thumbs under the rib cage. Breathe together and on the exhalation gently press inward and upward. Repeat this procedure, beginning at the center of the rib cage and working your way out to the periphery. This step is good for activating the liver, spleen, pancreas, and stomach. Repeat several times. (*See illustration top of next page.*)

14. Locate the point in the indented region at the bottom of the rib cage, about halfway between the center of the rib

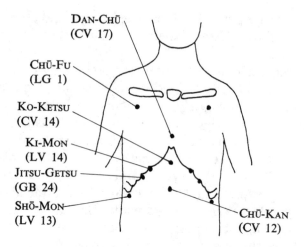

DAN-CHŪ
(CV 17)

CHŪ-FU
(LG 1)

KO-KETSU
(CV 14)

KI-MON
(LV 14)

JITSU-GETSU
(GB 24)

SHŌ-MON
(LV 13)

CHŪ-KAN
(CV 12)

cage and the periphery. This point, known as *Ki-Mon*, or Liver 14, is the *Bo*, or "gathering" point for the liver. The Bo points are the points on the front of the body where energy from the organs is discharged. They are complementary to the Yu, or entrance points along the bladder meridian on the back.

Use your thumbs to press and massage this point. This point energizes the liver and spleen. Oriental doctors also used this point to treat conditions such as gallstones, bronchitis, hepatitis, over-acid stomach, and diarrhea.

15. Locate the point at the bottom edge of the rib cage. This point, known as *Sho-Mon*, or Liver 13, is the gathering or Bo point for the spleen. It can be used to energize the liver and spleen. Oriental doctors also used it to treat water retention in the abdomen and arthritis of the chest.

Massage this point as described in the above step.

Further Refinements

As we saw in the previous chapter, there are Go and Gen points on the legs. Those on the front and side meridians can be massaged during the above steps. The Bo points, the places where energy gathers and is discharged from the body, are located on the front and can also be massaged.

The conception vessel, stomach, kidney, liver, and spleen meridians run along the front of the body and can also be massaged at this time, as can the gallbladder meridian on the side of the body. Massage these meridians with gentle thumb pressure.

Facial Massage

While the receiver is lying comfortably on the back, shift your position so that you are above the receiver's head. This will leave your hands free to massage the face. The facial massage can include the following:

1. Extend your hands forward so that your palms are resting lightly on the receiver's cheeks. Hold your hands in this position for about a minute, and breathe together with a relaxed and gentle rhythm.

2. Using your fingers, gently rub the cheeks up and down until they become warm. This sends energy to the lungs, energizing and activating them.

3. Ask the receiver to close his or her eyes and keep them closed during the next three procedures. Extend your hands forward and place both palms over the receiver's eyes. Keep them in this position for about thirty seconds and breathe in the same rhythm as the receiver. This energizes the regions around the eyes and helps relax tension and stress.

4. Use the index, middle, and ring fingers of both hands to press gently along the bony edge of the upper eye socket, moving from the inner to the outer corner of the eye. Repeat several times and then press the bone underneath the eye in the same manner. Do both eyes at the same time.

5. With the tips of the same three fingers, slowly and gently press the front of the eyeballs. Slowly press in and then quickly detach. Do both eyes at the same time and repeat about ten times to release stress and tension in the eyes. This procedure also helps calm the heart rhythm.

6. Use the thumb and index finger of your active hand to pinch the bridge of the nose and corners of the eyes. Push

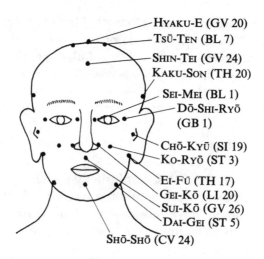

HYAKU-E (GV 20)
TSŪ-TEN (BL 7)
SHIN-TEI (GV 24)
KAKU-SON (TH 20)
SEI-MEI (BL 1)
DŌ-SHI-RYŌ (GB 1)
CHŌ-KYŪ (SI 19)
KO-RYŌ (ST 3)
EI-FŪ (TH 17)
GEI-KŌ (LI 20)
SUI-KŌ (GV 26)
DAI-GEI (ST 5)
SHŌ-SHŌ (CV 24)

deeply for about ten seconds and the quickly detach by pulling your fingers away. Repeat three to five times in order to relieve strain and fatigue in the eyes.

This region corresponds to the point, *Sei-Mei*, or Bladder 1. This is the beginning of the bladder meridian, and can be used to diagnose astigmatism, cataracts, and other eye disorders. It can also be used to treat headaches and problems in the kidneys and bladder.

7. With the fingertips of both hands, rub the sides of the nose up and down until it becomes warm. This activates the stomach, spleen, and pancreas, and helps stabilize the receiver's breathing.

8. Place the first four fingers of both hands on the area between the mouth and nose. Begin to massage this area with a gentle circular motion. Continue for about thirty seconds and the do the same thing below the mouth. Find the point in the middle of this region known as *Sui-Ko*, or Governing Vessel 26. Use your thumb or fingertips to press and release this point. This helps release tension in the face as a whole.

9. Find the point on both sides of the face next to the nostrils. This point is known as *Gei-Ko*, or Large Intestine 20. It is the end point of the large intestine meridian and can be used to treat toothache, facial paralysis, nose bleeding, and to help the receiver discharge stagnated mucus in the sinus or nasal region. Position the tips of both middle fingers on these

50

points. Use a circular motion to rub and massage the points for about a minute.

10. Position the tips of both middle fingers in the indented place in the middle of the cheeks, about a finger-width from the sides of the nose. Use a circular motion to rub and massage these points for about a minute. This relieves tension in the face caused by sinus congestion. This point is known as *Ko-Ryo* or Stomach 3. It is used to diagnose nasal disorders and to treat facial paralysis, toothache, and gum disease.

11. Find the point in the middle of the chin. This point is known as *Sho-Sho*, or Conception Vessel 24. It is the end point of the conception vessel and can be used to treat toothache, facial pain, and facial paralysis. Place your thumb or the tip of your middle finger on this point and massage for about thirty seconds.

12. Place the tips of the index, middle, and ring fingers of both hands under the lower jaw below the chin. (Your index fingers should be touching.) Press in and then release, and move your fingers up along the lower jaw, continuing to press and release, until you reach the ears.

13. Find the indented place a little more than halfway up the jawbone. This point is known as *Dai-Gei*, or Stomach 5. Insert the tips of your middle fingers in these points and massage with a circular motion. Stimulating this point helps energize the teeth and gums.

14. Locate the point where the ear meets the jaw. Known as *Ei-Fu*, or Triple Heater 17, this point can be used to treat ear and tooth disorders and to relieve tightness in the neck and shoulders. Massage this point as in the above step.

Further Refinements

Aside from the points mentioned above, there are other important points on the face. Study and incorporate these into your massage routine. Moreover, the regions of the face correspond to the internal organs and parts of the body. These correspondences provide the basis for traditional Oriental facial diagnosis and can be used during the facial massage.

Step 6
Concluding the Massage

To conclude the massage, place one hand lightly on the person's abdomen and the other lightly on the forehead. Breathe together for a minute or two, or until he or she is completely relaxed. Detach your hands by slowly raising them upward.

If the massage has been done properly, the receiver should feel relaxed yet energized. After you complete the massage, ask the receiver to remain in a resting position for about five minutes. Meanwhile, wash your hands in cold water to remove any excess energy that you may have picked up during the massage. With this, your basic massage is now complete. After the receiver has rested, ask how he or she feels. Then you can discuss the massage and make suggestions that can help the person improve his or her condition.

Once the basic massage technique has been mastered, feel free to experiment and continuously add new approaches to your practice. In this way, your massage will remain dynamic, and you will be able to develop your own original style.

Each massage will always be slightly different. The basic routine can serve as a general outline; however, it needs to be flexibly adapted to suit the needs of every person whom you treat. For example, in the morning or during the day, an active, stimulating massage is usually appropriate, while in the evening, a relaxing or calming massage would be suitable.

Similarly, you would massage a child differently than an elderly person, and a man differently than a woman. Also, since everyone's condition is unique, it is important to develop your sensitivity to energy. In this way, you can adjust your massage to suit the needs of the person you are treating. When you develop this intuitive ability and use it in conjunction with a centered, orderly technique, you are on your way to becoming a compassionate healer.

Step 7
Shiatsu Diagnosis

A skilled practitioner of Shiatsu is sensitive to energy. He or she is able to detect physical and energetic imbalances in the receiver and identify their causes. Many influences shape the balance of energy in the body, including activity, home and work environment, relationships, and general level of stress. However, among these, food is the most basic.

If your goal is to develop a genuine "feel" for energy and to use Shiatsu as a means to gain a deeper understanding of the cause of various conditions, it is important to avoid extremes and eat a balanced natural diet. This centers you and increases your sensitivity, and provides you with daily experience of the way in which diet affects health and well-being.

For the most part, the modern diet is based on extremes. Eggs, meat, cheese, chicken, and other animal foods have extremely yang energy. They produce constriction and tightening in the body, and cause heat and energy to flow inward, leading eventually to accumulation and blockage. Strong yang foods cause excess energy to build up inside the body. They also dull our sensitivity.

Foods such as spices, sugar, chocolate, tropical fruits, coffee, alcohol, and nightshade vegetables have the opposite effect. They have extremely yin or expansive energy, as do most drugs, medications, and food additives. When we eat spices, for example, capillaries at the surface of the body dilate, causing heat and energy to flow outward. This leads to an eventual dissipation and weakening of energy. Extremely yin foods cause energy to scatter and disperse, and interfere with our ability to detect energy from the outside.

A diet based on extremes disrupts the balance of energy and leads to various stages of disease. Basing the daily diet on whole grains, fresh local vegetables, beans and bean products, low-fat, white meat fish, seasonal fruits, and other whole natural foods promotes optimal vitality and sensitivity. These foods are energetically balanced, and do not block, scatter, or otherwise disrupt energy in the chakras, organs, cells, and meridians.

The Effects of Food

Shiatsu is a powerful tool for both diagnosis and treatment. When you give a massage, you mobilize your senses of touch, sight, hearing, and smell, together with your ability to perceive energy directly through your meridians. These senses can help you detect the underlying dietary and lifestyle causes of imbalance. Aside from making it possible to diagnose specific points, Shiatsu can be used to evaluate a person's condition as a whole. Sharing that information with the receiver can help him better understand the cause of his condition. Below are simple diagnostic signs that can help you identify dietary extremes when you give Shiatsu.

Saturated Fat and Cholesterol

Fat accounts for more than 40 percent of the average diet in America, mostly in the form of hard, saturated fat. Saturated fats are solid at room temperature, are yang in comparison to unsaturated vegetable oils. They are found in eggs, meat, cheese, chicken, yogurt, milk, butter, and other animal foods, and in many processed snack foods. As saturated fat accumulates in the blood vessels, organs, and tissues, the body becomes rigid and energy in the primary channel and chakras becomes blocked.

Saturated fat also accumulates below the skin, clogging

the pores and sweat glands and causing the skin to become hard and dry. This interferes with the movement of energy through the meridians. Animal foods are also the source of cholesterol, a substance that accumulates in the arteries and blood vessels, making them harder and less flexible.

What to Look for During Shiatsu:

- Inflexibility in the neck and other joints
- Tight overly expanded shoulders
- Hard dry skin
- Deeply etched wrinkles on the face, including deep vertical lines between the eyebrows, the area of the face that corresponds to the liver
- Hair loss in the center of the head
- Thick calluses on the bottoms of the feet or hands
- Dense body fat
- Distortion, discoloration, or unevenness on the nail of the large toe
- Overall tightness, hardness, or stagnation along the meridians

Animal Protein

Compared to the proteins found in plant foods, animal proteins are highly unstable. They break down into toxic bacteria and compounds such as uric acid and ammonia. These by-products accumulate in the kidneys and intestines, weakening their ability to discharge toxic excess. Consumption of too much animal protein leaches calcium and other minerals from the body, contributing to osteoporosis and weakening of the bones. Excess protein is discharged through the meridians and accumulates in the form of skin growths, discharges, and excess facial or body hair.

What to Look for During Shiatsu:

- Calluses on the bottoms of the feet or palms of the

hands
- Moles, warts, or other skin growths along the meridians, on the back, or on the face
- Excess facial or body hair
- An uneven skin texture
- Thin or depleted bones
- Dark circles around the eyes, in the area that corresponds to the kidneys and adrenal glands
- Pain or stagnation along the large intestine, small intestine, liver, or kidney meridians
- An unpleasant body odor

Simple Sugars

Simple sugars are made up of loose or fragmented molecules of glucose. They are yin in comparison to complex carbohydrates. The molecules in complex carbohydrates are fused into long chains. Simple sugars are found in foods such as candy, chocolate, cookies, honey, maple syrup, and in fruits, both temperate and tropical. Complex carbohydrates are found in whole grains, beans, vegetables, and sea vegetables, and are preferred for daily consumption. Simple sugars are rapidly absorbed and produce a quick rise in blood sugar levels. The pancreas then secretes insulin that causes excess sugar to be absorbed by the cells. Frequent consumption of simple sugars results in irregular metabolism—a rapid sugar "high" followed by a dip in energy as blood sugar drops.

The rapid absorption and burning of simple sugars in the body depletes energy in the chakras, meridians, and cells, and results in fatigue, tiredness, and a "burnt-out" feeling. Simple sugars also deplete minerals from the bloodstream, bones, and teeth, leading to overall weakening of the body.

What to Look for During Shiatsu:

- Puffiness or swelling of the facial features, especially the nose (which corresponds to the heart), and the lips (which correspond to the digestive organs)

- Overall puffiness or sagging of the skin
- An excess of soft body fat
- Freckles or large brown "age spots" (these frequently appear along the meridians)
- Redness or swelling at the tips of the fingers or toes
- Small white dots on the fingernails
- A reddish color on the nose (showing overexpansion of the heart); on the cheeks (showing overexpansion of the lungs); or in the face as a whole
- Extreme sensitivity to touch
- Coldness in the hands or feet

Excess Liquid

Drinking in excess expands and loosens cells and tissues and diminishes their ability to conduct energy. Drinking too much is often the result of consuming animal food and salt. Salt, which is yang, causes attraction to liquids which are yin. Animal foods contain plenty of fat which causes the body to retain heat, and this causes the attraction for ice-cold drinks. Excess liquid increases the volume of fluid in the circulatory system and causes the heart, kidneys, bladder, and sweat glands to overwork, leading to chronic fatigue, frequent urination, and excessive perspiration.

What to Look for During Shiatsu:

- Loose, flabby skin with a "washed out" appearance
- Eye bags (an indication of fluid retention in the kidneys)
- Moist or wet hands or feet
- Numerous horizontal wrinkles on the forehead
- Pain or swelling in the kidney region in the middle back
- Baldness caused by a receding hairline
- Pain when the point in the center of the palm (along the heart governor meridian) is pressed
- Coldness at the periphery of the body
- Malformation of the fifth toe (bladder meridian)

Poor Quality Salt

Processed snack foods, such as chips and pretzels, are very high in sodium, as are canned and fast foods, and many animal products. Salt, especially refined table salt or unrefined gray sea salt, is yang or contractive. It causes the tissues to constrict or tighten, and when taken excessively, diminishes energy in the chakras and meridians. It also contributes to fluid retention and can harden deposits of fat and cholesterol in the body. More balanced white sea salt contains many trace minerals, and is recommended for regular use in moderate amounts.

What to Look for During Shiatsu:

- Tight dry skin
- Coldness at the periphery of the body (caused by constriction of capillaries)
- Dark circles around the eyes
- A dark or yellowish complexion
- Tiny red dots on the skin or along the meridians
- Pain or tightness in the kidney region in the middle back
- Rigidity in the joints or body as a whole
- Swelling in the legs, ankles, or feet (caused by fluid retention)
- A tight, tense, or rigid personality

Chemicals, Additives, and Processed Foods

In comparison to whole natural foods, processed foods lack freshness, vitality, and energy. Eating them depletes energy in the chakras, meridians, and organs. Chemicals and additives accumulate in the organs, tissues, and cells, and weaken the charge of energy in the body. Fresh organic foods that are grown locally are preferred to artificially processed foods. Refined foods lack vitamins and minerals and disrupt the overall harmony of energy in the body.

What to Look for During Shiatsu:

- Skin with a stale or wilted look
- An uneven texture or color to the skin
- Pain in the kidney region in the middle back or along the kidney meridian
- Pain or swelling in the liver
- Pain along the liver meridian
- Deterioration in muscle tone
- Oversensitivity to touch, sound, smell, and other forms of environmental stimulation, such as in Environmental Illness (E.I.)

Giving Lifestyle Advice

While you are giving a massage, make a mental note of the points you wish to discuss with the receiver. For example, you may discover that certain organs, meridians, or points are tight, certain parts of the body are overly expanded, or that the energy in certain places is deficient. When you have finished the massage, discuss your observations with the receiver. Your goal should be to help the receiver gain a better understanding of his or her condition.

After presenting your evaluation, the next step is to explain the dietary and lifestyle causes of these conditions. For example, if the person you are treating has hard dry skin or moist hands or feet, you can mention that these signs are caused by too much saturated fat or too much liquid. If you discover tightness in the kidneys, inform the receiver that this is often due to too much salt, liquid, and fat.

The next step, after explaining the cause of important symptoms, is to explain to the receiver how he or she can change these conditions. If he or she is drinking too much coffee and fruit juice, for example, you can suggest a reduction or a change in the quality of beverages being consumed. In some cases, you may need to suggest that a person reduce the intake of animal food, stop eating chicken or cheese, or shift from simple to complex carbohydrates. The type of suggestions you make will depend on each person's unique condition and needs. In some cases, they could be minor—for example, reducing the intake of baked goods—while in others, more substantial changes could be necessary to restore optimal health.

Your suggestions can also include advice about activity and lifestyle. For example, one person may need to get more sleep in order to recharge their energy, while another may benefit from exercise and activity. Someone may need to reduce stress, while someone else may benefit from more challenging circumstances. One person may benefit from using natural fabrics and materials in the home, while another may need to shift from microwave to gas cooking. The dietary and lifestyle guidelines in the following section can help you in making appropriate recommendations.

By adding these steps, you begin to act as an educator who guides others toward health, happiness, and self-realization. You empower the people whom you treat by providing them with the knowledge they need to successfully manage their health. In this way, your practice of Shiatsu can evolve beyond therapy toward health education and preventive medicine.

Step 8
Developing Your Healing Power

Unlike the steps performed with a partner, the practices in this chapter must be done on your own. They help you develop the qualities needed to practice Shiatsu—vitality, strength, and stamina on the inside, and flexibility, sensitivity, and receptivity on the outside. They help make your condition strong yet peaceful, focused yet gentle, and increase your power to heal through touch.

It is important to remember that any form of touch involves the exchange of vibration. All matter, including that which comprises the body, is made up of energy. What we perceive as solid and tangible is actually made up of condensed units of vibrating energy. These are known scientifically as electrons, protons, and other subatomic particles. When you touch someone, your energy field and her energy field come into contact. There is actually no contact between one "solid" object and another. "Physical" contact is actually energetic contact.

The quality of your energy is determined by your thinking and lifestyle. Peaceful, healthy, and harmonious energy is immediately transferred to the receiver, making her more peaceful and harmonious. At the same time, if your energy is agitated, depressed, or stagnated, these qualities will also be transferred to the receiver. The strength of your healing power depends on your overall physical and emotional health, and these are, in turn, the product of the foods you eat, the type of activity you pursue, your home and work environment, and the quality of your relationships.

A Balanced Diet

A diet based on complex carbohydrates is ideal for developing the stamina and sensitivity required for Shiatsu. Complex carbohydrates are very low in fat and contain no cholesterol, both of which interfere with sensitivity to energy. They release their energy in a slow, steady manner, and help you maintain stamina and endurance. The general guidelines presented below can help you in selecting the most healthful foods. (For more detailed guidelines please refer to *Standard Macrobiotic Diet*, by Michio Kushi, One Peaceful World Press, 1992.)

Whole Cereal Grains Whole grains are nutritionally and energetically complete. They are composed largely of complex carbohydrates and increase your sensitivity, stamina, and endurance. They can be the principal food at each meal, and can comprise from 50 to 60 percent of your daily intake. Whole grains include brown rice, sweet brown rice, whole wheat berries, barley, millet, oats, and rye, as well as corn, buckwheat, and other botanically similar plants.

Whole grain products, such as cracked wheat, rolled oats, noodles, pasta, bread, baked goods, seitan (wheat meat), and other unrefined flour products may be included on occasion. However, please note that the energy in flour products is less strong than that in whole grains themselves.

Soups Soups are a hearty and nourishing way to prepare and serve vegetables, sea vegetables, beans, and whole grains. One or two small bowls of soup can be served daily, comprising about 5 to 10 percent of your daily intake. Soup broths can be seasoned with vegetable quality seasonings such as miso (naturally fermented soybean and grain puree) and tamari soy sauce (traditional, non-chemical soy sauce). Canned, packaged, or ready-made soups lack energy and are best avoided.

Vegetables About 25 to 30 percent of your daily intake can include fresh local vegetables prepared in a variety of ways, including steaming, boiling, baking, sauteing, pickling (without spices), salads, and marinades.

More centrally balanced vegetables for daily use include: green cabbage, kale, broccoli, cauliflower, collards, pumpkin, watercress, Chinese cabbage, bok choy, dandelion, mustard greens, daikon root and greens, scallion, onions, turnips, acorn squash, butternut squash, buttercup squash, burdock, carrots, and other seasonally available varieties. More extremely yin vegetables are best avoided or eaten only rarely. These include: potatoes, sweet potatoes, yams, tomatoes, eggplant, peppers, asparagus, spinach, beets, zucchini, and avocado. Mayonnaise and factory-made salad dressings are best avoided, as are vegetables imported from the tropics.

Beans, Bean Products, and Sea Vegetables About 5 to 10 percent of your daily intake can include cooked beans, bean products, and sea vegetables. Varieties such as azukis, chickpeas, and lentils are good for daily use, as are natural soybean products such as tofu, tempeh, and natto. Sea vegetables are a good source of minerals and include wakame, kombu, nori, hiziki, arame, and dulse.

Seasoning and Oil Naturally processed white sea salt can be used in seasoning, along with miso, tamari soy sauce, umeboshi and brown rice vinegar, fresh grated ginger, and other traditional items. Naturally processed, unrefined vegetable oil is recommended for daily cooking such as dark sesame seed oil. Kuzu is commonly used for sauces and gravies.

Condiments Condiments include gomashio (roasted sesame salt), roasted sea vegetable powders, umeboshi (pickled plums), tekka root vegetable powder, and others made from whole natural foods.

Pickles A small volume of non-spicy pickles, made at home or bought at the natural food store, can be eaten daily to aid in digestion of grains and vegetables.

Beverages Spring or well water are charged with energy from the earth and recommended for drinking, preparing tea, and cooking. Bancha twig tea (also known as *kukicha*) contains no caffeine and is ideal as a daily beverage, though roasted barley tea, and other grain-based teas, or traditional, non-stimulant herbal teas are fine for use.

Occasional Foods

Animal Food A small volume of low-fat, white-meat fish or seafood may be eaten a few times per week.

Seeds and Nuts Seeds and nuts, lightly roasted and salted with sea salt or seasoned with tamari soy sauce, may be enjoyed as occasional snacks.

Fruit Fruit may be eaten several times per week, preferably cooked or naturally dried, as a snack or dessert, provided the fruit grows locally or in a similar climate.

Dessert Occasional desserts, such as cookies, cake, pudding, pie, and other dishes can be made with naturally sweet foods such as apples, fall and winter squashes, azuki beans, chestnuts, or dried fruit, or can be sweetened with natural grain-based sweeteners such as rice syrup, barley malt, or amasake.

Foods to Minimize or Avoid

If you live in a temperate climate, avoiding or substantially reducing your intake of the following foods will greatly enhance your sensitivity to energy as well as your personal health:

• Meat, animal fat, eggs, poultry, dairy products (including butter, yogurt, ice cream, milk, and cheese), refined sugars, chocolate, molasses, honey, other simple sugars and foods treated with them, and vanilla.

• Tropical or semitropical fruits and fruit juices, soda, artificially flavored drinks and beverages, coffee, colored tea, distilled water, and aromatic or stimulant beverages.

• All artificially colored, preserved, sprayed, chemically treated, or genetically engineered foods. All refined and polished grains, flours, and their derivatives. Mass produced foods including canned, frozen, and irradiated foods. Hot spices, aromatic or stimulant foods, artificial vinegar, and strong alcoholic beverages.

The way we eat can be just as important as our choice of foods. Regularly scheduled meals are best. Snacking is best kept to a minimum so that it doesn't replace meals, while tea and other beverages can be enjoyed throughout the day as desired. Chewing is also important; try to chew each mouthful of food until it becomes liquid. The more you chew, the stronger your energy flow becomes. Eat whenever you feel hungry, but try to avoid eating at least three hours before bedtime. Food eaten before sleeping does not digest properly and can lead to indigestion and stagnation in the body. The most effective Shiatsu is given on a slightly empty stomach rather than after a big meal.

A Natural Lifestyle

Together with eating well, a variety of practices are recommended for health and well-being, and for re-establishing contact with the energy of our natural environment. Practices such as keeping physically active and using natural cooking utensils, fabrics, and materials in the home are especially recommended.

In the past, people lived in direct contact with natural energies and ate a more balanced natural diet. With each generation, we have gotten further from our roots in nature, and have experienced a corresponding decline in health. The suggestions presented below complement a balanced natural diet and can help make the flow of Ki through your chakras, meridians, and points more balanced and active.

•Try to get to bed before midnight and get up early in the morning.

•Try not to wear synthetic clothing or woolen articles directly against your skin. Wear cotton instead. Keep jewelry and accessories simple, natural, and graceful.

•Go outdoors in simple clothing every day. When the

weather permits, walk barefoot on the grass, the soil, or the beach. Go on regular outings, especially to beautiful natural areas.

•Try not to take long, hot baths or showers unless you have been consuming too much salt or animal food.

•Every morning or every night, scrub your body with a hot, moist towel until your circulation and energy flow become active. When a complete body scrub is not possible, at least do your hands and fingers, feet and toes. These areas are the most peripheral regions of the meridians and activate the inner regions of the organs.

•Use natural cosmetics, soaps, shampoos, and body care products.

•Keep as active as you can. Daily activities such as cooking and cleaning are excellent forms of exercise. Exercise programs such as yoga, marital arts, Do-In (self-massage), aerobics, and sports are also good. A daily half-hour walk is an especially good way to activate your energy and circulation.

•Try to minimize time spent in front of the television. Color TV, especially, emits unnatural radiation that can be physically and energetically draining.

•Switch from electric to gas cooking at the earliest opportunity. Microwave cooking is best avoided.

•Put many green plants throughout your home to freshen and enrich the air.

Centering Your Energy

Quieting the mind through meditation helps center your energy. Clearing the mind of unnecessary or unhelpful thoughts allows healing energy to flow smoothly. Meditation, including the simple regulation of breathing, can thus be a powerful tool in healing. The simple exercise that follows can be performed regularly to help you give effective Shiatsu.

1. Find a quiet place and sit in a relaxed and comfortable position. Yoga practices usually recommend the half-lotus position, but this can induce the tendency to hunch over. To

keep the spine straight while sitting in this position, you can sit on a pillow or cushion.

An even better way of sitting is to sit on the heels; that is, with the feet tucked under the legs so that the arches of the feet form a rounded place to sit in. The big toes can hold each other: one on top of the other. If you are not comfortable sitting on the floor, sitting in a chair is also fine.

2. The most effective and relaxing meditation is done when your posture is straight but relaxed. To straighten your posture, raise your arms up toward the ceiling and hold them there for a few moments. Then tilt your head so that you are looking up. Keep your head in this position for several seconds, and then lower your arms to their normal position at your side. Return your head to normal a moment later.

This simple stretching exercise straightens the spine and allows the energy of heaven and earth to flow smoothly through your body. Each of these steps can be done as a continuous sequence and the entire procedure can be repeated several times.

3. With your spine straight and your shoulders and elbows relaxed, place your hands in your lap with the palms facing up. Place your left hand, which corresponds to heaven, on top of your right, which corresponds to the earth.

4. Lift your thumbs upward and touch the tips of both thumbs together, forming an arc, or bridge. Your thumbs and index fingers should generally form a circle. This position creates unity and harmony between the the flow of heaven's and earth's forces on the left and right sides of the body.

5. Close your eyes and begin to breathe naturally and quietly. Breathe in a normal, relaxed manner. After making your breathing calm and quiet, begin to breathe deeply, centering your breath in the lower abdomen, or hara. As you breathe in, let your abdomen expand; and as you breathe out, let it contract.

6. While you are breathing in this manner, let your mind become quiet, relaxed, and free of distracting thoughts or images. Do not try to force distracting thoughts to go away but simply let them dissolve. It may help to concentrate on your breathing.

7. Sit this way for several minutes, breathing naturally and keeping your mind still and quiet. Keep your posture straight while allowing your body to relax completely.

8. To complete your meditation, slowly open your eyes and let your breathing return to normal. Then bring your consciousness back to a normal waking state.

Once the mind has been cleared of distraction, it is much easier to practice Shiatsu. A clear, peaceful mind makes it easier to maintain internal harmony and convey healthy, positive energy to the people you treat.

Meridian Charts

Lung Meridian
Energy flow: body to hand
Organ structure: yang (solid and compact)
Meridian energy: yin (subtle and less active)
Peak activity: 3–5 a.m.

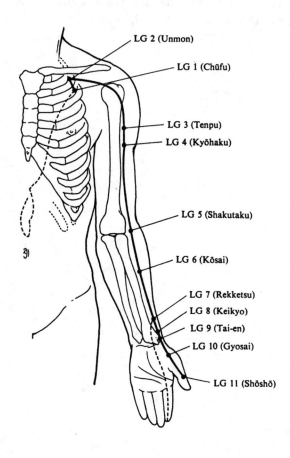

LG 2 (Unmon)
LG 1 (Chūfu)
LG 3 (Tenpu)
LG 4 (Kyōhaku)
LG 5 (Shakutaku)
LG 6 (Kōsai)
LG 7 (Rekketsu)
LG 8 (Keikyo)
LG 9 (Tai-en)
LG 10 (Gyosai)
LG 11 (Shōshō)

Heart Meridian

Energy flow: body to hand
Organ structure: yang
Meridian energy: yin
Peak activity: 11 a.m.–1 p.m.

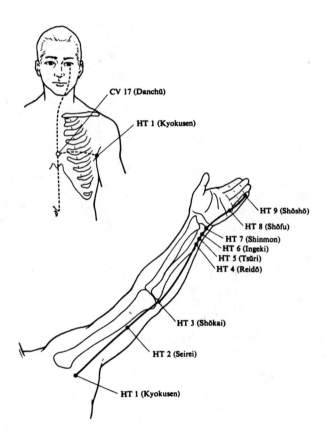

CV 17 (Danchū)

HT 1 (Kyokusen)

HT 9 (Shōshō)
HT 8 (Shōfu)
HT 7 (Shinmon)
HT 6 (Ingeki)
HT 5 (Tsūri)
HT 4 (Reidō)

HT 3 (Shōkai)

HT 2 (Seirei)

HT 1 (Kyokusen)

Large Intestine Meridian

Energy flow: hand to body
Organ structure: yin (hollow and expanded)
Meridian energy: yang (active)
Peak activity: 5–7 a.m.

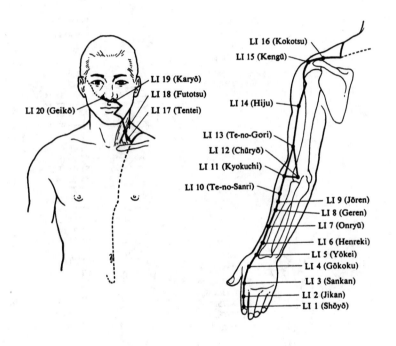

LI 16 (Kokotsu)
LI 15 (Kengū)

LI 19 (Karyō)
LI 18 (Futotsu)
LI 17 (Tentei)

LI 14 (Hiju)

LI 20 (Geikō)

LI 13 (Te-no-Gori)
LI 12 (Chūryō)
LI 11 (Kyokuchi)

LI 10 (Te-no-Sanri)

LI 9 (Jōren)
LI 8 (Geren)
LI 7 (Onryū)
LI 6 (Henreki)
LI 5 (Yōkei)
LI 4 (Gōkoku)
LI 3 (Sankan)
LI 2 (Jikan)
LI 1 (Shōyō)

Stomach Meridian

Energy flow: body to foot
Organ structure: yin
Meridian energy: yang
Peak activity: 7–9 a.m.

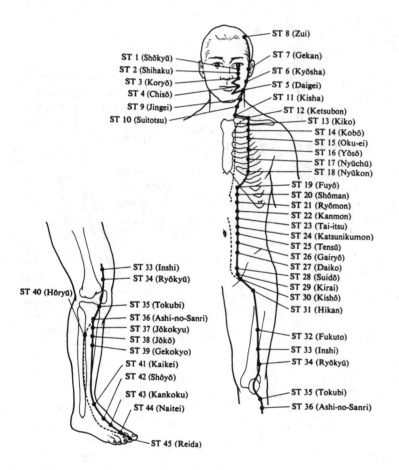

ST 8 (Zui)
ST 1 (Shōkyū)
ST 7 (Gekan)
ST 2 (Shihaku)
ST 6 (Kyōsha)
ST 3 (Koryō)
ST 5 (Daigei)
ST 4 (Chisō)
ST 11 (Kisha)
ST 9 (Jingei)
ST 12 (Ketsubon)
ST 10 (Suitotsu)
ST 13 (Kiko)
ST 14 (Kobō)
ST 15 (Oku-ei)
ST 16 (Yōsō)
ST 17 (Nyūchū)
ST 18 (Nyūkon)
ST 19 (Fuyō)
ST 20 (Shōman)
ST 21 (Ryōmon)
ST 22 (Kanmon)
ST 23 (Tai-itsu)
ST 24 (Katsunikumon)
ST 25 (Tensū)
ST 26 (Gairyō)
ST 33 (Inshi)
ST 27 (Daiko)
ST 34 (Ryōkyū)
ST 28 (Suidō)
ST 29 (Kirai)
ST 40 (Hōryū)
ST 30 (Kishō)
ST 35 (Tokubi)
ST 31 (Hikan)
ST 36 (Ashi-no-Sanri)
ST 37 (Jōkokyu)
ST 38 (Jōkō)
ST 32 (Fukuto)
ST 39 (Gekokyo)
ST 33 (Inshi)
ST 41 (Kaikei)
ST 34 (Ryōkyū)
ST 42 (Shōyō)
ST 43 (Kankoku)
ST 35 (Tokubi)
ST 44 (Naitei)
ST 36 (Ashi-no-Sanri)
ST 45 (Reida)

Spleen Meridian

Energy flow: foot to body
Organ structure: yang
Meridian energy: yin
Peak activity: 9–11 a.m.

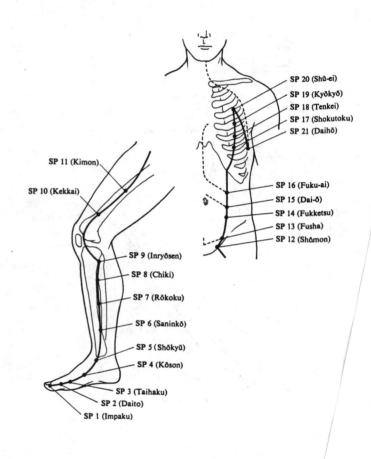

SP 20 (Shū-ei)
SP 19 (Kyōkyō)
SP 18 (Tenkei)
SP 17 (Shokutoku)
SP 21 (Daihō)
SP 11 (Kimon)
SP 16 (Fuku-ai)
SP 10 (Kekkai)
SP 15 (Dai-ō)
SP 14 (Fukketsu)
SP 13 (Fusha)
SP 12 (Shōmon)
SP 9 (Inryōsen)
SP 8 (Chiki)
SP 7 (Rōkoku)
SP 6 (Saninkō)
SP 5 (Shōkyū)
SP 4 (Kōson)
SP 3 (Taihaku)
SP 2 (Daito)
SP 1 (Impaku)

Small Intestine Meridian

Energy flow: hand to body
Organ structure: yin
Meridian energy: yang
Peak activity: 1–3 p.m.

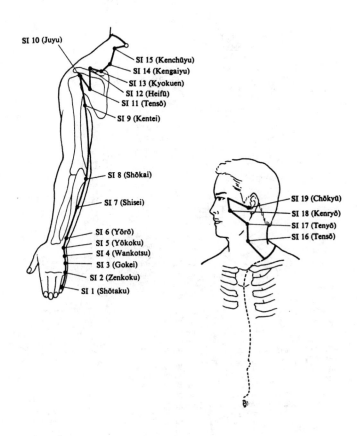

SI 10 (Juyu)

SI 15 (Kenchūyu)
SI 14 (Kengaiyu)
SI 13 (Kyokuen)
SI 12 (Heifū)
SI 11 (Tensō)

SI 9 (Kentei)

SI 8 (Shōkai)

SI 7 (Shisei)

SI 6 (Yōrō)
SI 5 (Yōkoku)
SI 4 (Wankotsu)
SI 3 (Gokei)
SI 2 (Zenkoku)
SI 1 (Shōtaku)

SI 19 (Chōkyū)
SI 18 (Kenryō)
SI 17 (Tenyō)
SI 16 (Tensō)

Bladder Meridian

Energy flow: body to foot
Organ structure: yin
Meridian energy: yang
Peak activity: 3—5 p.m.

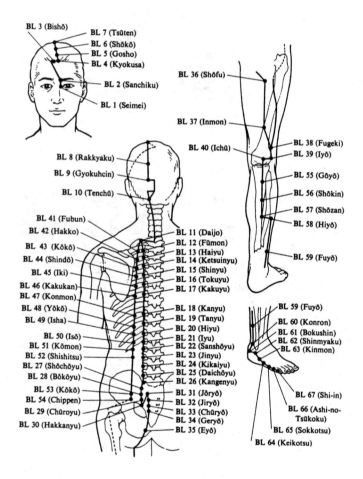

BL 3 (Bishō)
BL 7 (Tsūten)
BL 6 (Shōkō)
BL 5 (Gosho)
BL 4 (Kyokusa)
BL 2 (Sanchiku)
BL 1 (Seimei)

BL 36 (Shōfu)

BL 37 (Inmon)

BL 40 (Ichū)

BL 8 (Rakkyaku)
BL 9 (Gyokuhcin)
BL 10 (Tenchū)

BL 38 (Fugeki)
BL 39 (Iyō)
BL 55 (Gōyō)
BL 56 (Shōkin)
BL 57 (Shōzan)
BL 58 (Hiyō)

BL 41 (Fubun)
BL 42 (Hakko)
BL 43 (Kōkō)
BL 44 (Shindō)
BL 45 (Iki)
BL 46 (Kakukan)
BL 47 (Konmon)
BL 48 (Yōkō)
BL 49 (Isha)
BL 50 (Isō)
BL 51 (Kōmon)
BL 52 (Shishitsu)
BL 27 (Shōchōyu)
BL 28 (Bōkōyu)
BL 53 (Kōkō)
BL 54 (Chippen)
BL 29 (Chūroyu)
BL 30 (Hakkanyu)

BL 11 (Daijo)
BL 12 (Fūmon)
BL 13 (Haiyu)
BL 14 (Ketsuinyu)
BL 15 (Shinyu)
BL 16 (Tokuyu)
BL 17 (Kakuyu)
BL 18 (Kanyu)
BL 19 (Tanyu)
BL 20 (Hiyu)
BL 21 (Iyu)
BL 22 (Sanshōyu)
BL 23 (Jinyu)
BL 24 (Kikaiyu)
BL 25 (Daichōyu)
BL 26 (Kangenyu)
BL 31 (Jōryō)
BL 32 (Jiryō)
BL 33 (Chūryō)
BL 34 (Geryō)
BL 35 (Eyō)

BL 59 (Fuyō)

BL 59 (Fuyō)
BL 60 (Konron)
BL 61 (Bokushin)
BL 62 (Shinmyaku)
BL 63 (Kinmon)
BL 67 (Shi-in)
BL 66 (Ashi-no-Tsūkoku)
BL 65 (Sokkotsu)
BL 64 (Keikotsu)

Large Intestine Meridian

Energy flow: hand to body
Organ structure: yin (hollow and expanded)
Meridian energy: yang (active)
Peak activity: 5–7 a.m.

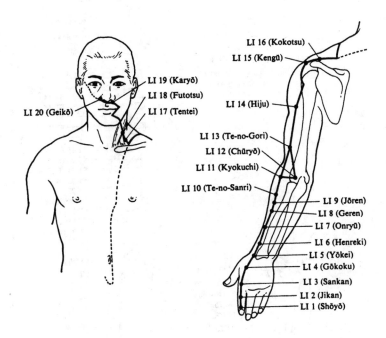

LI 16 (Kokotsu)
LI 15 (Kengū)
LI 14 (Hiju)
LI 13 (Te-no-Gori)
LI 12 (Chūryō)
LI 11 (Kyokuchi)
LI 10 (Te-no-Sanri)
LI 9 (Jōren)
LI 8 (Geren)
LI 7 (Onryū)
LI 6 (Henreki)
LI 5 (Yōkei)
LI 4 (Gōkoku)
LI 3 (Sankan)
LI 2 (Jikan)
LI 1 (Shōyō)

LI 19 (Karyō)
LI 18 (Futotsu)
LI 17 (Tentei)
LI 20 (Geikō)

Stomach Meridian

Energy flow: body to foot
Organ structure: yin
Meridian energy: yang
Peak activity: 7–9 a.m.

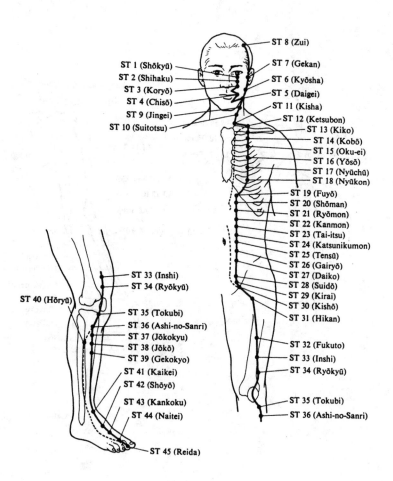

ST 8 (Zui)
ST 1 (Shōkyū)
ST 2 (Shihaku)
ST 3 (Koryō)
ST 4 (Chisō)
ST 9 (Jingei)
ST 10 (Suitotsu)
ST 7 (Gekan)
ST 6 (Kyōsha)
ST 5 (Daigei)
ST 11 (Kisha)
ST 12 (Ketsubon)
ST 13 (Kiko)
ST 14 (Kobō)
ST 15 (Oku-ei)
ST 16 (Yōsō)
ST 17 (Nyūchū)
ST 18 (Nyūkon)
ST 19 (Fuyō)
ST 20 (Shōman)
ST 21 (Ryōmon)
ST 22 (Kanmon)
ST 23 (Tai-itsu)
ST 24 (Katsunikumon)
ST 25 (Tensū)
ST 26 (Gairyō)
ST 27 (Daiko)
ST 28 (Suidō)
ST 29 (Kirai)
ST 30 (Kishō)
ST 31 (Hikan)

ST 33 (Inshi)
ST 34 (Ryōkyū)
ST 40 (Hōryū)
ST 35 (Tokubi)
ST 36 (Ashi-no-Sanri)
ST 37 (Jōkokyu)
ST 38 (Jōkō)
ST 39 (Gekokyo)
ST 41 (Kaikei)
ST 42 (Shōyō)
ST 43 (Kankoku)
ST 44 (Naitei)
ST 32 (Fukuto)
ST 33 (Inshi)
ST 34 (Ryōkyū)
ST 35 (Tokubi)
ST 36 (Ashi-no-Sanri)
ST 45 (Reida)

Spleen Meridian
Energy flow: foot to body
Organ structure: yang
Meridian energy: yin
Peak activity: 9–11 a.m.

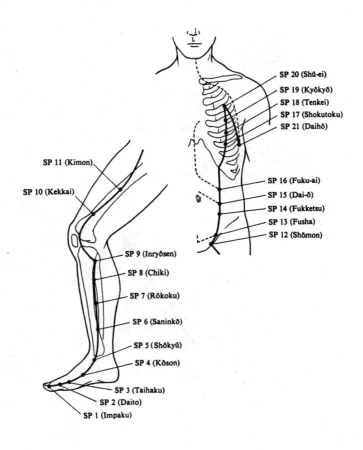

SP 20 (Shū-ei)
SP 19 (Kyōkyō)
SP 18 (Tenkei)
SP 17 (Shokutoku)
SP 21 (Daihō)

SP 11 (Kimon)

SP 10 (Kekkai)

SP 16 (Fuku-ai)
SP 15 (Dai-ō)
SP 14 (Fukketsu)
SP 13 (Fusha)
SP 12 (Shōmon)

SP 9 (Inryōsen)

SP 8 (Chiki)

SP 7 (Rōkoku)

SP 6 (Saninkō)

SP 5 (Shōkyū)
SP 4 (Kōson)

SP 3 (Taihaku)
SP 2 (Daito)
SP 1 (Impaku)

Heart Meridian

Energy flow: body to hand
Organ structure: yang
Meridian energy: yin
Peak activity: 11 a.m.–1 p.m.

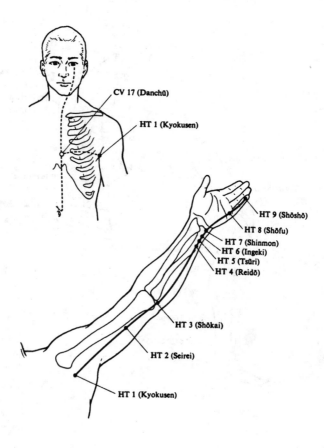

CV 17 (Danchū)

HT 1 (Kyokusen)

HT 9 (Shōshō)

HT 8 (Shōfu)

HT 7 (Shinmon)

HT 6 (Ingeki)

HT 5 (Tsūri)

HT 4 (Reidō)

HT 3 (Shōkai)

HT 2 (Seirei)

HT 1 (Kyokusen)

Small Intestine Meridian

Energy flow: hand to body
Organ structure: yin
Meridian energy: yang
Peak activity: 1–3 p.m.

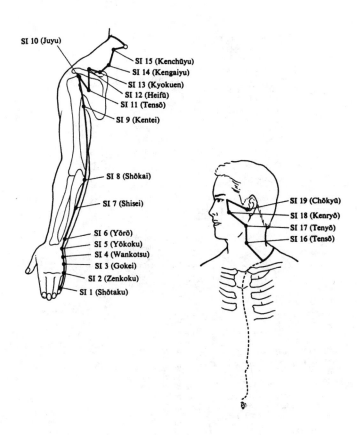

SI 10 (Juyu)

SI 15 (Kenchûyu)
SI 14 (Kengaiyu)
SI 13 (Kyokuen)
SI 12 (Heifû)
SI 11 (Tensô)

SI 9 (Kentei)

SI 8 (Shôkai)

SI 7 (Shisei)

SI 6 (Yôrô)
SI 5 (Yôkoku)
SI 4 (Wankotsu)
SI 3 (Gokei)
SI 2 (Zenkoku)
SI 1 (Shôtaku)

SI 19 (Chôkyû)
SI 18 (Kenryô)
SI 17 (Tenyô)
SI 16 (Tensô)

Bladder Meridian
Energy flow: body to foot
Organ structure: yin
Meridian energy: yang
Peak activity: 3—5 p.m.

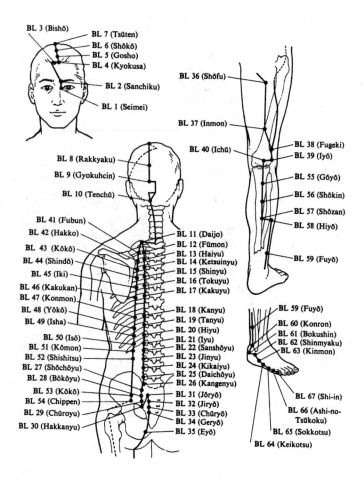

BL 3 (Bishō)
BL 7 (Tsūten)
BL 6 (Shōkō)
BL 5 (Gosho)
BL 4 (Kyokusa)
BL 2 (Sanchiku)
BL 1 (Seimei)
BL 36 (Shōfu)
BL 37 (Inmon)
BL 40 (Ichū)
BL 38 (Fugeki)
BL 39 (Iyō)
BL 8 (Rakkyaku)
BL 9 (Gyokuhcin)
BL 10 (Tenchū)
BL 55 (Gōyō)
BL 56 (Shōkin)
BL 57 (Shōzan)
BL 58 (Hiyō)
BL 41 (Fubun)
BL 42 (Hakko)
BL 43 (Kōkō)
BL 44 (Shindō)
BL 45 (Iki)
BL 46 (Kakukan)
BL 47 (Konmon)
BL 48 (Yōkō)
BL 49 (Isha)
BL 11 (Daijo)
BL 12 (Fūmon)
BL 13 (Haiyu)
BL 14 (Ketsuinyu)
BL 15 (Shinyu)
BL 16 (Tokuyu)
BL 17 (Kakuyu)
BL 59 (Fuyō)
BL 18 (Kanyu)
BL 19 (Tanyu)
BL 20 (Hiyu)
BL 21 (Iyu)
BL 22 (Sanshōyu)
BL 23 (Jinyu)
BL 24 (Kikaiyu)
BL 25 (Daichōyu)
BL 26 (Kangenyu)
BL 50 (Isō)
BL 51 (Kōmon)
BL 52 (Shishitsu)
BL 27 (Shōchōyu)
BL 28 (Bōkōyu)
BL 53 (Kōkō)
BL 54 (Chippen)
BL 29 (Chūroyu)
BL 30 (Hakkanyu)
BL 31 (Jōryō)
BL 32 (Jiryō)
BL 33 (Chūryō)
BL 34 (Geryō)
BL 35 (Eyō)
BL 59 (Fuyō)
BL 60 (Konron)
BL 61 (Bokushin)
BL 62 (Shinmyaku)
BL 63 (Kinmon)
BL 67 (Shi-in)
BL 66 (Ashi-no-Tsūkoku)
BL 65 (Sokkotsu)
BL 64 (Keikotsu)

Kidney Meridian
Energy flow: foot to body
Organ structure: yang
Meridian energy: yin
Peak activity: 5–7 p.m.

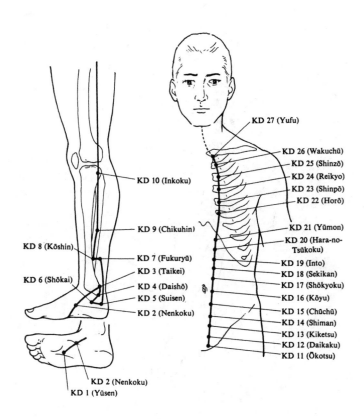

KD 27 (Yufu)

KD 26 (Wakuchū)
KD 25 (Shinzō)
KD 24 (Reikyo)
KD 23 (Shinpō)
KD 22 (Horō)

KD 10 (Inkoku)

KD 9 (Chikuhin)

KD 21 (Yūmon)
KD 20 (Hara-no-Tsūkoku)

KD 8 (Kōshin)

KD 7 (Fukuryū)
KD 3 (Taikei)
KD 4 (Daishō)
KD 5 (Suisen)
KD 2 (Nenkoku)

KD 6 (Shōkai)

KD 19 (Into)
KD 18 (Sekikan)
KD 17 (Shōkyoku)
KD 16 (Kōyu)
KD 15 (Chūchū)
KD 14 (Shiman)
KD 13 (Kiketsu)
KD 12 (Daikaku)
KD 11 (Ōkotsu)

KD 2 (Nenkoku)
KD 1 (Yūsen)

77

Heart Governor Meridian

Energy flow: body to hand
Physical function: yang
Meridian energy: yin
Peak activity: 7–9 p.m.

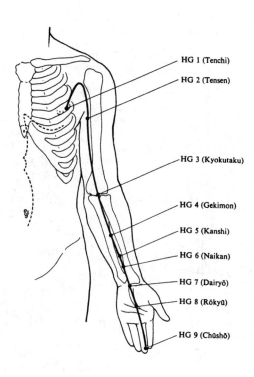

HG 1 (Tenchi)
HG 2 (Tensen)
HG 3 (Kyokutaku)
HG 4 (Gekimon)
HG 5 (Kanshi)
HG 6 (Naikan)
HG 7 (Dairyō)
HG 8 (Rōkyū)
HG 9 (Chūshō)

Triple Heater Meridian

Energy flow: hand to body
Physical function: yin
Meridian energy: yang
Peak activity: 9—11 p.m.

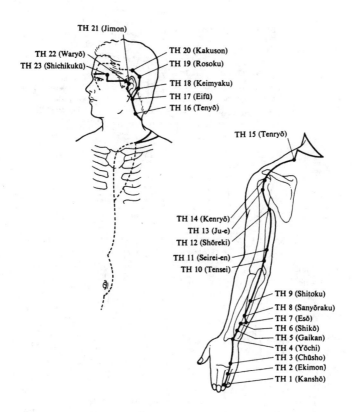

TH 21 (Jimon)

TH 22 (Waryō)
TH 23 (Shichikukū)

TH 20 (Kakuson)
TH 19 (Rosoku)

TH 18 (Keimyaku)
TH 17 (Eifū)
TH 16 (Tenyō)

TH 15 (Tenryō)

TH 14 (Kenryō)
TH 13 (Ju-e)
TH 12 (Shōreki)
TH 11 (Seirei-en)
TH 10 (Tensei)

TH 9 (Shitoku)
TH 8 (Sanyōraku)
TH 7 (Esō)
TH 6 (Shikō)
TH 5 (Gaikan)
TH 4 (Yōchi)
TH 3 (Chūsho)
TH 2 (Ekimon)
TH 1 (Kanshō)

Gallbladder Meridian

Energy flow: body to foot
Organ structure: yin
Meridian energy: yang
Peak activity: 11 p.m.–1 a.m.

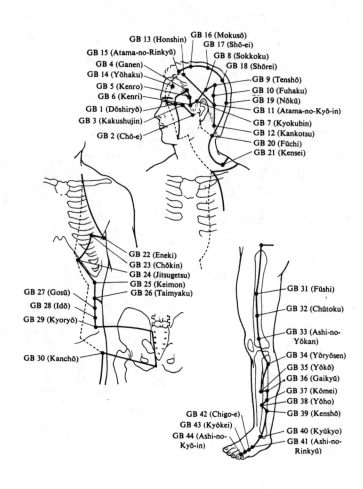

GB 13 (Honshin)
GB 16 (Mokusō)
GB 17 (Shō-ei)
GB 15 (Atama-no-Rinkyū)
GB 4 (Ganen)
GB 8 (Sokkoku)
GB 14 (Yōhaku)
GB 18 (Shōrei)
GB 5 (Kenro)
GB 9 (Tenshō)
GB 6 (Kenri)
GB 10 (Fuhaku)
GB 19 (Nōkū)
GB 1 (Dōshiryō)
GB 11 (Atama-no-Kyō-in)
GB 3 (Kakushujin)
GB 7 (Kyokubin)
GB 12 (Kankotsu)
GB 2 (Chō-e)
GB 20 (Fūchi)
GB 21 (Kensei)

GB 22 (Eneki)
GB 23 (Chōkin)
GB 24 (Jitsugetsu)
GB 25 (Keimon)
GB 27 (Gosū)
GB 26 (Taimyaku)
GB 28 (Idō)
GB 29 (Kyoryō)
GB 31 (Fūshi)
GB 32 (Chūtoku)
GB 33 (Ashi-no-Yōkan)
GB 30 (Kanchō)
GB 34 (Yōryōsen)
GB 35 (Yōkō)
GB 36 (Gaikyū)
GB 37 (Kōmei)
GB 38 (Yōho)
GB 42 (Chigo-e)
GB 39 (Kenshō)
GB 43 (Kyōkei)
GB 44 (Ashi-no-Kyō-in)
GB 40 (Kyūkyo)
GB 41 (Ashi-no-Rinkyū)

Liver Meridian

Energy flow: foot to body
Organ structure: yang
Meridian energy: yin
Peak activity: 1–3 a.m.

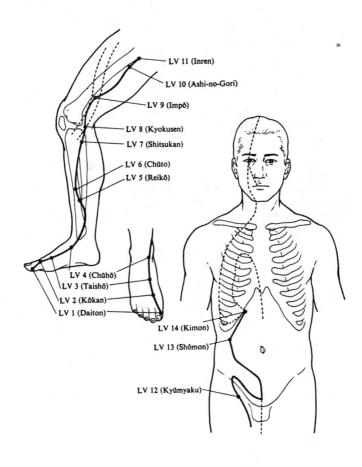

LV 11 (Inren)

LV 10 (Ashi-no-Gori)

LV 9 (Impō)

LV 8 (Kyokusen)

LV 7 (Shitsukan)

LV 6 (Chūto)

LV 5 (Reikō)

LV 4 (Chūhō)

LV 3 (Taishō)

LV 2 (Kōkan)

LV 1 (Daiton)

LV 14 (Kimon)

LV 13 (Shōmon)

LV 12 (Kyūmyaku)

Yu Points and Bo Points

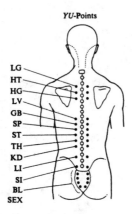

YU-Points

LG
HT
HG
LV
GB
SP
ST
TH
KD
LI
SI
BL
SEX

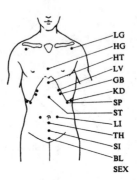

BO-Points

LG
HG
HT
LV
GB
KD
SP
ST
LI
TH
SI
BL
SEX

LG—Lungs
HT—Heart
HG—Heart Governor (Energy Circulation)
LV—Liver
GB—Gallbladder
SP—Spleen and Pancreas
ST—Stomach

TH—Triple Heater (Energy and Heat
   Metabolism)
KD—Kidneys
LI—Large Intestine
SI—Small Intestine
BL-SEX—Bladder and Sexual functions

Sei, Gen, and Go Points

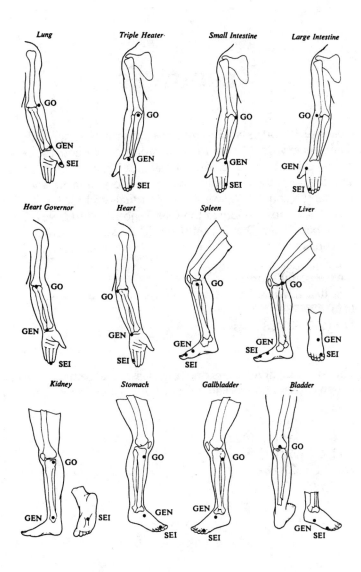

Resources

One Peaceful World is an international information network and friendship society devoted to the realization of one healthy, peaceful world. Activities include educational and spiritual tours, assemblies and forums, international food aid and development, and publishing. Membership is $30/year for individuals and $50 for families and includes a subscription to the One Peaceful World Newsletter and a free book from One Peaceful World Press. For further information, contact:

One Peaceful World
Box 10, Becket, MA 01223
(413) 623–2322
Fax (413) 623–8827

The Kushi Institute offers ongoing classes and seminars including Shiatsu classes and workshops. For information, contact:

Kushi Institute
Box 7, Becket MA 01223
(413) 623–5741
Fax (413) 623–8827

Recommended Reading

1. Esko, Edward. *Healing Planet Earth* (One Peaceful World Press, 1992).

2. Esko, Edward. *Notes from the Boundless Frontier* (One Peaceful World Press, 1992).

3. Esko, Edward. *The Pulse of Life* (One Peaceful World Press, 1994).

4. Esko, Wendy. *Introducing Macrobiotic Cooking* (Japan Publications, 1978).

5. Esko, Wendy. *Macrobiotic Cooking for Everyone* (with Edward Esko, Japan Publications, 1980).

6. Esko, Wendy. *Rice Is Nice* (One Peaceful World Press, 1995).

7. Faulkner, Hugh. *Physician Heal Thyself* (One Peaceful World Press, 1992).

8. Harris-Bonham, Jack. *Medicine Men: A Play about George Ohsawa* (One Peaceful World Press, 1993).

9. Jack, Alex. *Inspector Ginkgo, The Macrobiotic Detective* (One Peaceful World Press, 1994).

10. Jack, Alex. *Let Food Be Thy Medicine* (One Peaceful World Press, 1994).

11. Jack, Alex. *Out of Thin Air: A Satire on Owls and Ozone, Beef and Biodiversity, Grains and Global Warming* (One Peaceful World Press, 1993).

12. Jack, Gale and Alex. *Amber Waves of Grain: American Macrobiotic Cooking* (Japan Publications, 1992).

13. Kushi, Aveline. *Aveline Kushi's Complete Guide to Macrobiotic Cooking* (with Alex Jack, Warner Books, 1985).

14. Kushi, Aveline, with Wendy Esko. *Aveline Kushi's Wonderful World of Salads* (Japan Publications, 1989).

15. Kushi, Aveline, with Wendy Esko. *The Changing Seasons Cookbook* (Avery Publishing Group, 1985).

16. Kushi, Aveline, with Wendy Esko. *Diet for Natural Beauty* (Japan Publications, 1991).

17. Kushi, Aveline, with Wendy Esko. *The Good Morning Macro-*

17. Kushi, Aveline, with Wendy Esko. *The Good Morning Macrobiotic Breakfast Book* , (Avery Publishing Group, 1991).

18. Kushi, Aveline, with Wendy Esko. *The Macrobiotic Cancer Prevention Cookbook* (Avery Publishing Group, 1988).

19. Kushi, Aveline, with Wendy Esko. *Macrobiotic Family Favorites* (Japan Publications, 1987).

20. Kushi, Aveline, with Wendy Esko. *The New Pasta Cuisine* (Japan Publications, 1992).

21. Kushi, Aveline, with Wendy Esko. *The Quick and Natural Macrobiotic Cookbook* (Contemporary Books, 1989).

21. Kushi, Michio. *AIDS and Beyond* (with Alex Jack, One Peaceful World Press, 1995).

23. Kushi, Michio. *Basic Home Remedies* (One Peaceful World, 1994).

24. Kushi, Michio. *The Book of Macrobiotics* (with Alex Jack, Japan Publications, revised edition, 1986).

25. Kushi, Michio. *The Cancer-Prevention Diet* (with Alex Jack, St. Martin's Press, 1983; revised and updated edition, 1993).

26. Kushi, Michio. *Diet for a Strong Heart* (with Alex Jack, St. Martin's Press, 1985).

27. Kushi, Michio. *Forgotten Worlds* (with Edward Esko, One Peaceful World Press, 1992).

28. Kushi, Michio. *The Gospel of Peace: Jesus's Teachings of Eternal Truth* (with Alex Jack, Japan Publications, 1992).

29. Kushi, Michio. *Healing Harvest* (with Edward Esko, One Peaceful World Press, 1994).

30. Kushi, Michio. *Holistic Health Through Macrobiotics* (with Edward Esko, Japan Publications, 1993)

31. Kushi, Michio. *Nine Star Ki* (with Edward Esko, One Peaceful World Press, 1991).

32. Kushi, Michio. *One Peaceful World* (with Alex Jack, St. Martin's Press, 1986).

33. Kushi, Michio. *Other Dimensions: Exploring the Unexplained* (with Edward Esko, Avery Publishing Group, 1991).

34. Kushi, Michio. *The Philosopher's Stone* (with Edward Esko, One Peaceful World Press), 1994.

35. Kushi, Michio. *Spiritual Journey* (with Edward Esko, One Peaceful World Press), 1994.

36. Kushi, Michio. *The Teachings of Michio Kushi* (with Edward Esko, One Peaceful World Press, 1993).

37. Kushi, Michio, with Aveline Kushi *Raising Healthy Kids* (with Wendy and Edward Esko, Avery Publishing Group, 1994).

38. Lalumiere, Guy. *Macobiotic Home Food Processing*, One Peaceful World Press, 1993).

39. Sudo, Hanai. *Fire, Water, Wind* (One Peaceful World Press, 1992).

For a free catalog of macrobiotic books available by mail order, please write One Peaceful World Press, Box 10, Becket, MA 01223 or telephone (413) 623-2322.

About the Authors

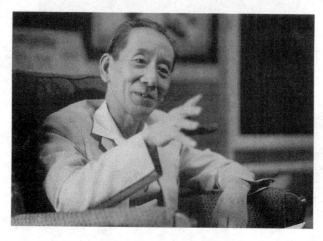

Michio Kushi, leader of the internantional macrobiotic community, was born in Janap in 1926, studied international relations and law at Tokyo University, and came to the United States in 1949. Devoted to the cause of world peace, he and his wife, Aveline, introduced modern macrobiotics to North America. Over the years, he has lectured and given seminars on diet and health, philosophy and culture, spiritual practice and ecology, to medical professionals, government officials, and individuals and families around the world, guiding thousands of people to greater health and happiness. Founder and president of the Kushi Foundation and One Peaceful World and author of numerous books, he maintains a busy international travel schedule and makes his home in Brookline, Massachusetts.

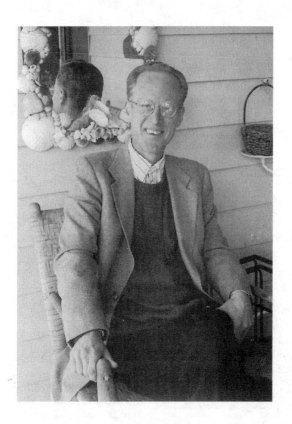

Edward Esko began macrobiotic studies with Michio Kushi in 1971 and for twenty years has taught macrobiotic philosophy throughout the United States and Canada, as well as in Western and Eastern Europe, South America, Asia and the Far East. He has lectured on modern health issues at the United Nations in New York and is on the faculty of the Kushi Institute in Becket, Mass. He is the author of *Healing Planet Earth*, *Notes from the Boundless Frontier*, and *The Pulse of Life*, and has co-authored or edited several popular books with Michio Kushi including *Holistic Health Through Macrobiotics*. He lives with his wife, Wendy, and their eight children in the Berkshires.

Index

Note: Points used in Basic Shiatsu are listed in boldface.

Basic Macrobiotics

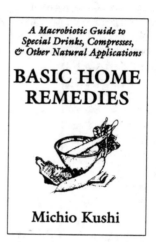

A Guide to Balanced Eating with Endless Variety and Satisfaction **Standard Macrobiotic Diet** Michio Kushi	*A Macrobiotic Guide to Special Drinks, Compresses, & Other Natural Applications* **BASIC HOME REMEDIES** Michio Kushi

Michio Kushi's Basic Introduction to Diet and Health Care

Available at Bookstores and Natural Food Stores or
By Mail Order from the Publisher:

One Peaceful World Press
Box 10
Becket, MA 01223
(413) 623-2322
Fax (413) 623-8827

Please send $5.95 per copy of *Standard Macrobiotic Diet* and $6.95 for *Basic Home Remedies*, plus $2.00 postage. Make check or money order payable to One Peaceful World (in U.S. funds drawn on a U.S. bank or send Visa/Mastercard # and expiration date.

Basic Cooking

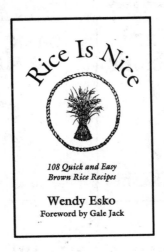

Rice Is Nice

*108 Quick and Easy
Brown Rice Recipes*

Wendy Esko
Foreword by Gale Jack

Wendy Esko's Introduction to Macrobiotic Cooking

Available at Bookstores and Natural Food Stores or
By Mail Order from the Publisher:

One Peaceful World Press
Box 10
Becket, MA 01223
(413) 623-2322
Fax (413) 623-8827

Please send $8.95 plus $2.00 postage per copy. Make check or
money order payable to One Peaceful World (in U.S. funds drawn
on a U.S. bank or send Visa/Mastercard # and expiration date.